Clinical Considerations in Perioperative Nursing

Preventive Aspects of Care

Edwina A. McConnell, RN, BS, MS, PhD

Consultant-Medical and Surgical Nursing
Formerly Clinical Director — Surgical Nursing
Madison General Hospital, Madison, Wisconsin

Clinical Considerations in Perioperative Nursing

Preventive Aspects of Care

J. B. LIPPINCOTT COMPANY   Philadelphia

London   Mexico City   New York   St. Louis   São Paulo   Sydney

Acquisitions Editor: Diana Intenzo
Sponsoring Editor: Eleanor Faven
Manuscript Editor: Lorraine D. Smith
Indexer: Betty Herr Hallinger
Design Director: Tracy Baldwin
Design Coordinator: Susan Hess Blaker
Production Manager: Kathleen P. Dunn
Production Coordinator: Ken Neimeister
Compositor: Digitype
Printer/Binder: R. R. Donnelley & Sons Company

3 5 6 4 2

Library of Congress Cataloging-in-Publication Data

McConnell, Edwina A.
  Clinical considerations in perioperative nursing.

  Includes bibliographies and index.
  1. Surgical nursing.   2. Surgery — Complications
and sequelae.   I. Title.   [DNLM: 1. Intraoperative
Complications — prevention & control — nurses' instruction.
2. Postoperative Complications — prevention & control —
nurses' instruction. 3. Preoperative Care — nurses'
instruction. 4. Surgical Nursing. WY 161 M478c]
RD99.M384 1987   617'.91'0024613   86-15403
ISBN 0-397-54494-4

The author and publisher have exerted every effort to
ensure that drug selection and dosage set forth in this text
are in accord with current recommendations and practice at
the time of publication. However, in view of ongoing
research, changes in government regulations, and the
constant flow of information relating to drug therapy and
drug reactions, the reader is urged to check the package
insert for each drug for any change in indications and
dosage and for added warnings and precautions. This is
particularly important when the recommended agent is a
new or infrequently employed drug.

To Abbie Ina Phinney
and Elwyn Carl McConnell
with Love and Thanks.
Without you none of this would
have been possible!

Foreword

Recently, a friend shared with me scenarios from her daughter's postoperative experience. It was a tale of poor nursing care. The friend concluded that "they should have *known* better." Although that phrase is used so frequently in our culture that its impact is diluted, in the case of my friend and her daughter it pinpoints the problem. The nurse(s) lacked essential knowledge and the patient did not receive quality perioperative nursing care.

Some authors/lecturers would lead health professionals to conclude that quality is no longer an issue; they identify the bottom line as *cost*. Cost containment is in; quality is out. The blame for this situation is placed on the insurance/reimbursement system, together with other social trends. Is it true that quality care is a concern of the past? I think not. I think the public will demand quality care and demand it in the context of reasonable cost. Americans are growing in sophistication regarding quality health care. They have seen statistics relating to regional differences in costs, in frequency of surgical procedures, and in length of hospital stay, as examples. They have also learned that the health status of the general public is not reflected in these statistics; the statistics are instead a reflection of preferences by health professionals. My observations lead me to conclude that we are entering an era when quality in health care delivery will be an expectation and an era in which the public will have a voice in determining health care outcome standards.

How do the two issues identified in the preceding paragraphs relate? Is there a relationship between knowledge and quality practice? If so, is the knowledge of the health professional likely to be subject to greater scrutiny in the years ahead? Although some nurses and some non-nurses think knowledge is less important for nurses than other traits such as experience, ability to follow orders, and a pleasant personality, most nurses and the general public appreciate the complex and extensive knowledge base required for professional nursing practice. Indeed, knowledge is essential to quality nursing care.

And how do these thoughts relate to this particular book, "Clinical Considerations in Perioperative Nursing"? They relate as follows. First, the author presents a clear picture of the relationship between knowledge and practice. Each chapter reinforces the link between knowledge and practice and also delineates the extensive knowledge base needed for perioperative nursing.

Perioperative nursing, even that part considered "technical," is vividly presented as a scientifically grounded practice. Second, quality care is of primary concern. The individual, the family, educational, psychosocial, and physiological dimensions of care, prevention, and continuity are components of the framework surrounding practice. The focus from beginning to end is quality as reflected in patient outcomes. In addition, the reader of this book will see nurses presented as critical to quality patient outcomes and as deliberative, reflective practitioners.

In this book, Edwina McConnell shares her vision of perioperative nursing care in which the patient and critical thinking are central. She presents a readable analysis and synthesis of the body of knowledge basic to quality in perioperative nursing practice.

I wish my friend's daughter had received perioperative nursing care from nurses with this knowledge base and view of nursing.

Carol A. Lindeman, RN, PhD, FAAN

Preface

Experience without theory is blind but theory without experience is
mere intellectual play.

—Kant

Perioperative nursing practice focuses on the "individual experiencing
surgical intervention." * It considers the "physiological, social and behavioral
problems resulting from or affecting the individual's response and/or adaptation to surgical intervention" * and is based on the basic principles of medical-
surgical nursing.

The successful outcome of a patient's perioperative experience hinges
upon the nurse who manages his care. Nurses care for and work with the
patient and his family throughout the perioperative period. They coordinate
his care and work with physicians and other health care professionals to ensure
a complication-free perioperative experience.

The perioperative nursing period is comprised of three phases: preoperative, intraoperative, and postoperative. As the diagram on the next page illustrates, these phases are linked together and build upon each other. Additionally, the perioperative period is inextricably linked to the nursing process.
Each phase of the perioperative period corresponds to a phase of the nursing

*American Nurses' Association Division on Medical-Surgical Nursing Practice and
Association of Operating Room Nurses: Standards of Perioperative Nursing Practice, p 3. Kansas City, MO, American Nurses' Association, 1981.

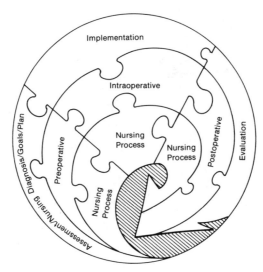

The interrelation of the perioperative nursing period and the nursing process.

process, while the nursing process is a part of each phase of the perioperative period. These various pieces fit together like those of a puzzle. The completed puzzle is a picture of an individual who has experienced a complication-free perioperative period.

The preoperative phase of the perioperative period involves not only patient assessment, identification of nursing diagnoses, and the derivation of goals, but also the development of a care plan. The plan is put into effect in the implementation phase and evaluated in the postoperative phase.

Each phase of the perioperative period incorporates the nursing process. The overall goal of the preoperative phase is to identify factors that increase the patient's risk of surgery and to prepare the patient physically and emotionally for surgery. The nurse identifies nursing diagnoses from assessment data, derives goals, and develops, implements, and evaluates the plan.

The general goal of the intraoperative phase is to ensure an uneventful surgical procedure, while protecting the patient from injury. Thus, the nurse assesses the patient and combines these data with those gleaned in the preoperative phase. She identifies nursing diagnoses, establishes goals, and implements and evaluates the plan. Additionally, she implements plans developed preoperatively that meet the patient's continuing needs.

The overall goal of the postoperative phase is to discharge the patient to home or to another health care facility, while ensuring continuity of care. Thus, the nurse assesses the patient and combines these data with those gathered throughout the pre- and intraoperative phases. She identifies nursing diagnoses from which she derives goals and then establishes, implements, and evaluates a plan of care.

Prevention of perioperative complications and nursing interventions that attain this goal are the focus of this book. Therefore, the chapters in Section 1, "The Preoperative Phase," focus on the physiology of stress, preoperative patient assessment, and patient preparation. Chapter 1 describes not only the physiological events of the stress response, but also nursing interventions that support the body's protective mechanisms and prevent the development of complications resulting from the stress response. Chapter 2 is devoted to preoperative patient evaluation, while Chapter 3 focuses on preparing the patient physically and emotionally for surgery. Preoperative assessment and preparation are the foundation for nursing care throughout the patient's hospitalization and planning for discharge.

Section 2 "The Intraoperative Phase," deals with the patient's experience from the time that he arrives in the operating room until he arrives in the postanesthesia recovery room. Chapter 4 discusses patient positioning, Chapter 5 explores anesthesia and its adjuncts, and Chapter 6 focuses on intraoperative techniques. Events of the preoperative phase contribute to an uneventful intraoperative phase, and events of the pre- and intraoperative phases contribute to a complication-free recovery and discharge.

Section 3, "The Postoperative Phase," begins with the patient's arrival in the postanesthesia recovery room and covers his care through discharge. Chapter 7 describes the patient's experience in the postanesthesia recovery room. This chapter, together with those in Section 2, is designed to provide the nurse on a surgical unit with an overview of the patient's experiences in the operating and postanesthesia recovery rooms. This is extremely important because the patient's intra- and immediate postoperative experiences affect his postoperative nursing care needs. Chapter 8 is devoted to avoiding or at least minimizing potential postoperative complications. Therefore, the pathophysiology of various complications, contributing factors, nursing strategies for prevention, and both medical and nursing therapies are presented. Chapter 9 is included in Section 3 because, even though planning for discharge begins when the patient is admitted, the goal is achieved in the postoperative period.

Nursing, the skillful art of caring, is both an art and a science. The skillful practitioner knowledgeably combines both practice and theory. Nurses caring for patients on surgical units frequently need information quickly, but then later wish for more in-depth information. These needs, combined with the fact that nursing *is* both an art and a science, determined the manner in which the content of this book is presented. Information that nurses need to know quickly is presented in tables, lists, forms, figures, and charts. The knowledge that provides the basis for this information is presented in narrative form. Therefore, a staff nurse can find the information that she needs quickly and still have in-depth knowledge readily available.

This book is written for the registered professional nurse working with surgical patients. Upper level students caring for surgical patients and other nurses interested in the comprehensive care of surgical patients will find this book useful. Presentation of the content presupposes an understanding of anatomy, physiology, basic physical assessment skills, the nursing process, and the *Standards of Perioperative Nursing Practice*. Procedures used in the art and science of perioperative nursing are not presented. Each nursing unit has a procedure manual to which readers are directed if they have questions about a specific procedure.

Throughout this book the professional registered nurse is referred to as "she" and the patient as "he." This choice of pronouns is not meant to be sexist but was chosen for ease and clarity in presentation.

Colleagues and friends who reviewed the manuscript and offered constructive comments are: Ann Digmann, RN; Cheryl Eller, RN; Louise M. Juliani, RN, MS; Ellen K. Murphy, MS, JD, CNOR; Gary E.D. Oldenburg, MD; Colleen Pfeiffer, MS, CCRN; Judith K. Sands, RN, EdD, and Mary F. Zimmerman, RN, MS. They, as well as Diana Intenzo, Carol E. Smith, RN, PhD, Sherry VanGorder, and James F. Welch offered welcome words of encouragement. To all of you I say, "Thank you!"

Edwina A. McConnell

What Is A Patient?*

The patient is the most important person in the hospital.

The patient is not dependent upon us — we are dependent upon him.

The patient is not an interruption of our work — he is the purpose of it.

The patient is not an outsider to our business — he is our business!

The patient is a person and not a statistic.

He has feelings, emotions, prejudices, and wants.

It is our business to SATISFY him.

*Seen on a bulletin board at the Wellington Polytechnic School of Nursing, Wellington, New Zealand.

Contents

Clinical Considerations in Perioperative Nursing

Preventive Aspects of Care

Section 1
The Preoperative Phase

The success of an operative procedure may well depend on the care exercised in preparing the patient.

—Norma A. Metheny, William D. Snively, Jr.

1 | The Physiology of Stress

All of the significant battles are waged within the self.

The perioperative period contains a number of potential stressors. These include a disease necessitating surgery; trauma, or trauma associated with the surgery itself; anesthesia; inadequate fluids, nutrients, and oxygen, and anger, frustration, and fear. While not every surgical patient perceives a potential stressor as a stressor, perception of any stimuli as stressful activates certain mechanisms or responses. These responses, in turn, are associated with certain physiological effects. Throughout the perioperative period the nurse intervenes to support the protective mechanisms and to prevent the development of complications.

| The Stress Response

Stress occurs within the body as a result of internal or external stimuli. When perceived as stressors, these physical or psychological stimuli provoke a generalized nonspecific response. That is, the response is the same regardless of the precipitating event. Usually the body's response does not eliminate the stressor, but rather contains or modifies it until it is alleviated.

The nervous and endocrine systems work together in order to respond to stressors and to maintain a stable internal environment. Perception of stressors causes activation of the sympathetic-adrenal medullary mechanism, the pituitary-adrenocortical mechanism, and the renin-angiotensin axis. Listed below are the components of the nervous and endocrine systems, including their respective hormones, that are involved in the stress response.

Parts of the Nervous and Endocrine Systems Involved in the Stress Response

The hypothalamus:

    Secretes corticotropin-releasing hormone (CRH)

    Secretes growth hormone-releasing factor (GHRF)

    Secretes thyrotropin-releasing hormone (TRH)

    Produces antidiuretic hormone (ADH)

The medulla oblongata:

    Transmits motor fibers from brain to spinal cord and sensory fibers from spinal cord to brain

    Contains collections of nerves that deal with vital functions

The sympathetic nervous system:

    Augments functions necessary to life and inhibits unnecessary functions

The adrenal medulla:

    Synthesizes and releases epinephrine

    Synthesizes and releases norepinephrine

The pituitary gland:

    Secretes adrenocorticotropic hormone (ACTH)

    Stores and releases antidiuretic hormone (ADH)

    Secretes growth hormone (GH)

    Secretes thyroid-stimulating hormone (TSH)

The adrenal cortex:

    Secretes glucocorticoids

    Secretes mineralocorticoids

The thyroid gland:

    Synthesizes and secretes thyroxine (T_4)

    Synthesizes and secretes triiodothyronine (T_3)

The renal juxtaglomerulus apparatus:

    Renin-angiotensin axis

| **The Nervous System**

The Hypothalamus and the Medulla Oblongata

The hypothalamus plays a significant role in regulating pituitary function. It collects and integrates signals from diverse sources, funnels them to the pituitary, and stimulates the release of several hormones including adrenocorticotropic hormone, growth hormone, and thyroid hormone. Nuclei on the hypothalamus also synthesize antidiuretic hormone, which is stored for release in the posterior pituitary.

The medulla oblongata is the enlarged portion of the spinal cord in the cranium after it enters the foramen magnum. This lower portion of the brain stem contains ascending and descending tracts. It transmits motor fibers from the brain to the spinal cord and sensory fibers from the spinal cord to the brain. In addition, it contains collections of nerves that deal with vital functions such as respiration, circulation, and special senses.

Perception of a stessor causes the body to increase the production and release of adrenal cortical hormones and catecholamines. For example, an increase or decrease in the blood level of oxygen, carbon dioxide, water, or sodium stimulates the hypothalamus either directly or indirectly via the medulla oblongata. Once stimulated, the hypothalamus activates the endocrine system, while the medulla oblongata activates the autonomic nervous system. Either the hypothalamus or the medulla oblongata stimulates the sympathetic-adrenal medullary mechanism and parts of the endocrine system, both of which are involved in the body's response to stressors.

The Sympathetic-Adrenal Medullary Mechanism

The autonomic nervous system has two major subdivisions: the sympathetic nervous system and the parasympathetic nervous system. It operates at a subconscious level and controls many functions of the internal organs, such as action of the heart and glandular secretion. Although mainly activated by centers in the spinal cord, brain stem, and hypothalamus, the autonomic nervous system often operates via visceral reflex arcs. That is, sensory signals enter the centers of the cord, brain stem, or hypothalamus, and these in turn send appropriate reflex responses to control the activities of the visceral functions.

The general organization of the sympathetic and parasympathetic nervous systems is illustrated in Figures 1-1 and 1-2, respectively. Because sympathetic fibers have many branches, stimulation of almost any portion of the system causes the entire system to respond. Complete stimulation of the sympathetic nervous system inhibits those functions not essential to life, while augmenting essential functions. The effects on different visceral functions caused by stimulation of the sympathetic and parasympathetic nervous systems are listed in Table 1-1.

In stressful situations the sympathetic nervous system focuses on sup-

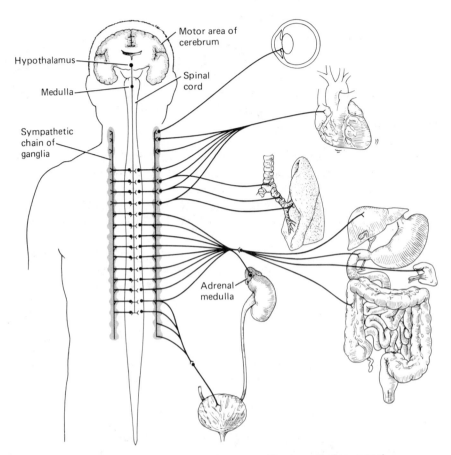

Figure 1-1. Distribution of sympathetic nerves. The hypothalamus and medulla direct impulses to sympathetic nerves that originate in the thoracic and lumbar regions of the spinal cord. Preganglionic sympathetic neurons pass from the spinal cord to ganglia, where they synapse. Then, postganglionic sympathetic neurons pass to the organs innervated.

portive activities such as increasing the heart and respiratory rates and mobilizing glucose from glycogen. Conversely, the parasympathetic nervous system focuses on conservative and restorative functions.

Catecholamines

The catecholamines — epinephrine and norepinephrine — are neurotransmitters whose absence would seriously compromise the body's stress response. They mediate peripheral sympathetic nervous system activity and are an essential element of the stress response.

The adrenal medullae synthesize both epinephrine and norepinephrine, and activation of the sympathetic nervous system initiates their release. As soon as they are released into the circulating blood, they are carried to all body tissues. Epinephrine, the key hormone in the fight or flight stress response, is produced only in the adrenal medullae. On the other hand, norepinephrine is produced both in the adrenal medullae and at adrenergic (sympathetic) nerve synapses throughout the body. It is released directly when the sympathetic nervous system is stimulated.

The effects of the circulating catecholamines released by the adrenal medullae resemble those effects caused by direct sympathetic stimulation, and

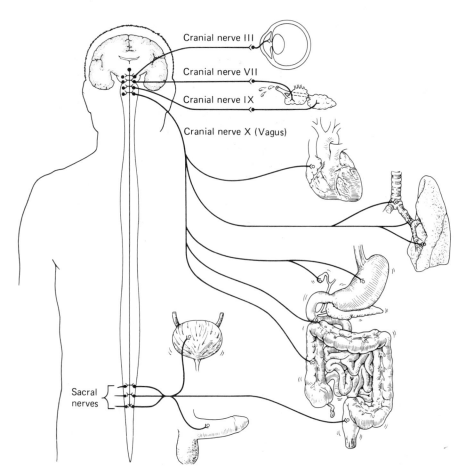

Figure 1-2. Distribution of parasympathetic nerves. Some parasympathetic neurons originate in the midbrain and medulla, where they join in forming certain cranial nerves. Other parasympathetic neurons originate in the sacral part of the spinal cord. Preganglionic neurons synapse in ganglia near the effector organs or synapse in the organs themselves. Postganglionic neurons are short.

Table 1-1
Autonomic Effects on Various Organs of the Body

Organ	Effect of Sympathetic Stimulation	Effect of Parasympathetic Stimulation
Eye: Pupil	Dilated	Constricted
Ciliary muscle	Slight relaxation	Contracted
Glands: Nasal Lacrimal Parotid Submaxillary Gastric Pancreatic	Vasoconstriction and slight secretion	Stimulation of thin, copious secretion (containing many enzymes for enzyme-secreting glands)
Sweat glands	Copious sweating (cholinergic)	None
Apocrine glands	Thick, odoriferous secretion	None
Heart: Muscle	Increased rate Increased force of contraction	Slowed rate Decreased force of atrial contraction
Coronaries	Dilated (β_2); constricted (α)	Dilated
Lungs: Bronchi	Dilated	Constricted
Blood vessels	Mildly constricted	? Dilated
Gut: Lumen	Decreased peristalsis and tone	Increased peristalsis and tone
Sphincter	Increased tone	Relaxed
Liver	Glucose released	Slight glycogen synthesis
Gallbladder and bile ducts	Relaxed	Contracted
Kidney	Decreased output	None
Bladder: Detrusor	Relaxed	Excited
Trigone	Excited	Relaxed
Penis	Ejaculation	Erection
Systemic blood vessels: Abdominal	Constricted	None
Muscle	Constricted (adrenergic α) Dilated (adrenergic β) Dilated (cholinergic)	None
Skin	Constricted	None
Blood: Coagulation	Increased	None
Glucose	Increased	None
Basal metabolism	Increased up to 100%	None
Adrenal cortical secretion	Increased	None
Mental activity	Increased	None
Pilorector muscles	Excited	None
Skeletal muscle	Increased glycogenolysis Increased strength	None

From Guyton AC: Textbook of Medical Physiology, 7th ed, p 691. Philadelphia, WB Saunders, 1986 the former enhance the action of the latter. However, the effects of the circulating catecholamines last longer than those caused by direct sympathetic stimulation. This is because the circulating catecholamines are removed from the blood more slowly than those released at the adrenergic nerve synapses.

Epinephrine and norepinephrine affect metabolism through glycogenolysis (the conversion of glycogen to glucose) in the liver and skeletal muscle and through mobilization of fatty acids. They increase the force and rate of cardiac contraction as well as the excitability of the myocardium. Circulating epinephrine and norepinephrine cause increased mental acuity, inhibition of the gastrointestinal and genitourinary tracts, pupillary dilation, and bronchiolar relaxation. Pupillary dilation allows better distance vision, and bronchiolar relaxation decreases airway resistance. Epinephrine causes dilation of the vessels of the liver and skeletal muscle, while norepinephrine causes vasoconstriction in most organs. As a result, blood is shunted toward exercising muscles, the heart, and the brain. Organs critical to fight or flight receive adequate substrate for energy production.

Epinephrine increases the basal metabolic rate and in this regard is 10 times more potent than norepinephrine. By increasing the basal metabolic rate, epinephrine increases the activity and excitability of the entire body. Additionally, epinephrine increases the rate of other metabolic activities.

Epinephrine stimulates glycogenolysis while simultaneously impeding glycogen synthesis. It also converts skeletal muscle glycogen to lactic acid that is transported to the liver and converted to new glucose. Epinephrine stimulates gluconeogenesis (the formation of glucose from molecules that are not themselves carbohydrates, such as from amino acids, lactate, and the glycerol portion of fats). While stimulating glucagon secretion, epinephrine concurrently inhibits insulin secretion. These actions help restore plasma glucose and its delivery to the central nervous system. At the same time, epinephrine activates adipose tissue lipase. This increases plasma-free fatty acids, their oxidation in muscle and liver, and ketogenesis. When secreted in response to stressors, epinephrine is a diabetogenic hormone; that is, its actions induce hyperglycemia and ketosis.

To differentiate the effects of epinephrine and norepinephrine on receptor cells, two distinct receptor catecholamine sites have been identified. They are alpha-receptors and beta-receptors. Located primarily in the precapillary sphincters of smooth muscles of blood vessels, alpha-receptors mediate vasoconstriction. Beta-receptors are located primarily in the heart, coronary arteries, liver, lungs, and brain, and mediate vasodilation.

Epinephrine affects cardiovascular functioning because it directly stimulates both α- and β-adrenergic receptors. Stimulation of cardiac β_1-adrenergic receptors causes an increase in cardiac rate and contractile force.

While the effects of norepinephrine are qualitatively identical to epinephrine, significant quantitative differences have been noted. Most significantly, norepinephrine less strongly stimulates β-adrenergic receptors on vascular smooth muscle. Therefore, it tends to constrict all vascular beds and to increase peripheral vascular resistance. The hypertension that results from the intense peripheral vasoconstriction leads to baroreceptor activation and reflex slowing of the heart. Consequently, cardiac output may be reduced. Table 1-2 identifies some actions of catecholamines that are α- and β-receptor mediated.

Table 1-2
Some Actions of Catecholamines

β-Receptor mediated (Epinephrine > norepinephrine)	α-Receptor mediated (Norepinephrine > epinephrine)
↑ Glycogenolysis	↑ Gluconeogenesis
↑ Lipolysis and ketosis	
↑ Calorigenesis	
↓ Glucose utilization	
↑ Insulin secretion	↓ Insulin secretion
↑ Glucagon secretion	
↑ Muscle K$^+$ uptake	
↑ Arteriolar dilation (muscle)	↑ Arteriolar vasoconstriction (splanchnic, renal, cutaneous, genital)
↑ Cardiac contractility (β_1)	
↑ Heart rate (β_1)	
↑ Cardiac conduction velocity (β_1)	
↑ Muscle relaxation (gastrointestinal, urinary, bronchial [β_2])	↑ Sphincter contraction (gastrointestinal, urinary) Sweating ("adrenergic") Dilation of pupils
↑ Renin secretion	↑ Growth hormone secretion
↑ Parathyroid hormone secretion ↑ Thyroid hormone secretion	

From Genuth SM: The adrenal glands. In Berne RM, Levy MN (eds): Physiology, p 1064. St. Louis, CV Mosby, 1983

Results of Sympathetic-Adrenal Medullary Stimulation

Stimulation of the sympathetic-adrenal medullary mechanism results in many physiological changes. Summarized on the opposite page, these changes help the body deal with stressors. Total stimulation augments the functions essential to life, while suppressing the unessential functions.

| The Endocrine System

The second system involved in the body's response to stressors is the endocrine system, specifically the pituitary-adrenocortical mechanism. This mechanism refers to the relationship between the hypothalamus, the anterior pitui-

Physiological Results of Sympathetic-Adrenal Medullary Stimulation

Cardiac rate and contractile force increase

Arterial pressure increases

Blood flow to active muscles increases with a concurrent decrease in blood flow to organs that are not needed for rapid activity

The skeletal muscles tense

Muscle strength increases

The skin is pale and moist

The rate of blood coagulation increases

Respiratory rate and depth increase

Bronchioles dilate

The cellular metabolic rate increases throughout the body

The concentration of blood glucose increases

Glycolysis in the muscles increases

Mental activity and alertness increase

Peristalsis decreases

The pupils dilate

tary gland, and the adrenal cortex, as well as to the roles played by their respective hormones. These include corticotropin releasing hormone (CRH), adrenocorticotropic hormone (ACTH), aldosterone, antidiuretic hormone (ADH), growth hormone (GH), and the thyroid hormones.

The Pituitary-Adrenocortical Mechanism

CRH and ACTH

Stressors such as surgery, trauma, infections, anxiety, and fear excite the hypothalamus, causing it to secrete corticotropin releasing hormone (CRH). This hormone is carried to the anterior pituitary gland where it induces secretion of ACTH that effects the release of large quantities of glucocorticoids. Cortisol accounts for at least 95% of the glucocorticoid activity of the adrenocortical secretions, and corticosterone and cortisone account for the other 5%.

The glucocorticoid secretion initiates a series of metabolic events aimed at relieving the damaging nature of the stressor. Direct feedback of the cortisol to the hypothalamus and anterior pituitary gland stabilizes its concentration. Normally, increased levels of CRH and ACTH inhibit further release, but in a stressful situation glucocorticoid secretion continues.

ACTH not only effects the release of glucocorticoids, but also increases secretion of mineralocorticoids. These adrenocortical steroids cause sodium conservation and potassium excretion by affecting the ion transport in the kidney cells. Aldosterone is the primary and most potent naturally occurring mineralocorticoid. It primarily regulates electrolytes (minerals) in the extra-cellular fluid.

Glucocorticoids.   The primary effect of the glucocorticoids is to raise blood glucose levels. In so doing, they alter the body's internal environment. Because they affect the metabolism of carbohydrates, proteins, and fats, the glucocorticoids cause catabolism and an anti-insulin effect. Their catabolic effects require decreased insulin, and they suppress insulin secretion while stimulating the production of glucagon. Together with glucagon and the catecholamines, glucocorticoids facilitate gluconeogenesis and increase the rate of glycogen synthesis as much as 6 to 10 times. Therefore, glucose is available at a time when it is or may be lacking in the diet. In addition, by increasing protein breakdown and decreasing its synthesis, glucocorticoids facilitate mobilization of amino acids from muscle. Low-molecular-weight nitrogen compounds are available for collagen synthesis in wound healing, and injured tissues are provided with the amino acids needed for the synthesis of other substances necessary to cell life.

The increased blood levels of glucocorticoids also help stabilize the body's internal environment by affecting sodium and water balance. Sodium reabsorption increases, volume expands, and potassium is excreted. The increased excretion of potassium occurs because glucocorticoid production increases the rate of muscle catabolism.

By influencing catecholamines, glucocorticoids also help combat stressors. They increase the effects and synthesis of catecholamines that help maintain adequate blood pressure and heart rate.

While many of the effects of glucocorticoid production are adaptive, some are not. For example, the increased circulating glucocorticosteroids cause a decrease in circulating lymphocytes, eosinophils, and basophils, and a decrease in macrophage activity. The increased circulating glucocorticoids depress inflammation and enhance the spread of infection.

Corticosteroid levels increase rapidly during stress. Plasma cortisol levels begin rising before surgery because of fear and apprehension. The plasma level rises quickly during surgery and for several hours postoperatively. In the absence of postoperative complications, the level returns to normal in about 3 days. Some research suggests that women normally have a higher plasma cortisol level postoperatively than men. Persistent stress causes the level to remain elevated for weeks or months.

When measuring plasma cortisol levels, it is very important to note the time at which the blood sample is drawn because glucocorticoid secretion follows a circadian pattern. The secretory rates of CRH, ACTH, and cortisol are high early in the morning but low in the late evening. The early morning elevation drops about 10 A.M., increases again about 2 P.M., and gradually decreases until 10 P.M. A 24-hour cyclic alteration in the hypothalamic signals that cause cortisol secretion are responsible for this pattern. When a person changes his sleeping habits, the cycle changes accordingly.

Aldosterone.   Secretion of this major mineralocorticoid increases in the stress response. High levels of ACTH may stimulate its secretion as does an increase in the potassium ion concentration of the extracellular fluid. However, the renin-angiotensinogen system is the major stimulus.

When the macula densa of the kidney (cells near the glomerulus) senses diminished renal blood flow or decreased blood sodium levels, it instructs the juxtaglomerular apparatus to release renin. Circulating catecholamines, which stimulate the juxtaglomerular apparatus, are a significant factor in renin release, especially with stress.

Renin acts on its substrate angiotensinogen, a serum protein, to form angiotensin I. A second enzyme in the lungs converts angiotensin I to angiotensin II that stimulates the adrenal cortex to secrete aldosterone. Angiotensin II is a vasoconstrictor that is 50 times as potent as norepinephrine. Therefore, in addition to stimulating the adrenal cortex, angiotensin II acts directly on renal arterioles, causing them to constrict. This decreases both the glomerular filtration rate and the reabsorption of sodium and water, and increases the supporting plasma and interstitial volume. Aldosterone's support of plasma and interstitial fluid volume, together with the release of angiotensin, helps maintain adequate circulating intravascular volume and the perfusion of vital organs. Angiotensin II plays a significant role in supporting the blood pressure of preoperative patients who are volume depleted, either because of poor intake, nasogastric suction, chronic diuretic therapy, or fever.

In addition to stimulating the reabsorption of sodium and water, aldosterone affects electrolyte metabolism. It causes the excretion of potassium, ammonium, and magnesium ions. Sodium is exchanged in the distal tubules for potassium and hydrogen ions.

This transient hyperaldosteronism produces the acid urine typical in the surgical patient. In addition to being acidic, the urine is high in potassium, low in sodium, and contributes to alkalemia that is common postoperatively. Urinary sodium in the early postoperative period is always below 40 mEq/liter and is often below 10 mEq/liter. Urinary sodium is a useful clinical measure of renal function because a value of 40 mEq/liter or less indicates renal dysfunction or acute tubular necrosis.

When the patient is no longer stressed and the renal plasma flow has returned to normal, the secretion of aldosterone stops abruptly and the kidney releases sodium and water. This diuretic phase occurs 3 to 4 days postoperatively. However, if the stress persists, so also do the effects of the aldosterone.

Antidiuretic Hormone

Antidiuretic hormone (ADH), also known as vasopressin, is produced in the hypothalamus and then is stored in and released from the posterior pituitary. It is released in response to changes in the body's internal environment such as increased osmolality, preoperative water deprivation, decreased vascular volume and blood pressure, and other stressors including pain, fever, many drugs, and possibly narcotic administration. By acting on the distal renal tubules and collecting ducts to reabsorb water, ADH causes increased blood volume and the excretion of concentrated urine.

A proportionate relationship exists between the volume depletion associated with trauma or surgery and the amount and persistence of the antidiuretic effects observed in the postoperative or posttraumatic state. A minimal reduction in volume causes a minimal release of antidiuretic hormone. A severe or persistent reduction in volume causes a prolonged and greater release of the hormone. Parameters indicating the extent and duration of the stress include urine volume and plasma and urine osmolality.

Growth Hormone

The anterior pituitary secretes growth hormone (somatotropin) under the direction of the hypothalamus. The latter releases growth hormone releasing factor (GHRF) that suppresses the release of somatostatin and stimulates the release of growth hormone. By mobilizing fatty acids and increasing fatty acid oxidates, growth hormone helps maintain adequate energy. Through gluconeogenesis, growth hormone spares protein catabolism and actually leads to increased protein synthesis. In addition, growth hormone decreases the peripheral use and uptake of glucose, impedes glucose tolerance, increases glucagon retention, and has antiinsulin properties. Hyperglycemia is the net action of growth hormone.

Thyroid Hormones

Secretion of the thyroid hormones is governed by the hypothalamus. Physiologic stressors trigger the hypothalamus to secrete thyrotropin releasing hormone (TRH) that in turn stimulates the anterior pituitary gland to secrete thyroid stimulating hormone (TSH) or thyrotropin. Secretion of TSH causes increased synthesis and secretion of thyroxine (T4) and triiodothyronine (T3) as well as an increased basal metabolic rate. These hormones help maintain a stable internal environment by keeping the temperature constant and the energy supply adequate. In addition, thyroxine seems to enhance the body's responsiveness to epinephrine. Epinephrine is thought to be more efficient in short-term stress, while thyroxine is more efficient in prolonged stress.

Results of Pituitary-Adrenocortical Stimulation

Stimulation of the pituitary-adrenocortical mechanism results in many physiological changes. Summarized on the opposite page, these changes are aimed at maintaining a stable internal environment.

| Preventive Nursing Interventions

Knowledge of the physiological effects of stress enables the nurse to intervene throughout the perioperative period. She supports the body's protective mechanisms and prevents complications that may develop as a result of the

Physiological Results of Pituitary-Adrenocortical Stimulation

Glomerular filtration rate decreases

Reabsorption of sodium and water increases

Blood volume increases

Urine output decreases

Urine specific gravity and osmolality increase

Urine is acidic, low in sodium, and high in potassium

Potassium, ammonium, and magnesium ions are excreted

Blood glucose levels are elevated

Levels of fatty acids and protein are increased

Insulin secretion is decreased

Protein catabolism increases

The body's defense mechanism is lowered

Inflammatory response is lowered

physiological effects of stress. She also attempts to prevent any additional stressors such as trauma, superimposed infection, anxiety, fear, pain, noise, and bright lights because the extent and severity of stimuli affect the intensity of the stress response.

Attempts are made to maintain the patient's normal 24-hour cycle of sleeping and waking. This makes it possible to predict low cortisol levels and therefore to avoid major stressors at a time when the body is least able to cope with them. The patient's care plan is individualized and prehospital sleep/wake patterns are closely approximated.

The stress response is a hypermetabolic state, and since the body is already using additional energy because of its increased metabolic rate, the patient needs rest. Activities or events that increase the body's metabolic rate are avoided. For example, the patient is kept comfortably warm, not hot and not cold. Increased body temperature not only increases the body's metabolic rate, as does shivering, but also counterbalances the arteriolar constriction needed to ensure an adequate blood supply to the vital organs.

Other nursing interventions can minimize the stress response. These include being thoughtful, considering the patient's preferences, providing emotional support, and increasing the continuity and consistency of care by limiting the number of nursing staff. Comfort measures such as backrubs, position changes, and back support are also important. They help alleviate anxiety, as well as generalized muscle tension, muscle aches, and headaches.

Table 1-3 summarizes the major physiological effects of stress. It also

Table 1-3
The Physiological Effects of Stress and Nursing Interventions To Avoid Potential Complications

Effect	Pathophysiology	Symptoms	Possible Untoward Effects	Nursing Interventions
Hypermetabolism	Catecholamine release leads to activation of the sympathetic nervous system, which causes: 1. Increased cardiac output 2. Increased energy secondary to glyconeogenesis and use of body stores	Increased blood pressure, pulse, and respiration; increased blood sugar, glycosuria; increased alertness; dilated pupils	Patients with cardiovascular or pulmonary disease may be unable to meet increased oxygen needs or to support circulatory demands of hypermetabolism. Diabetics may be unable to metabolize increased glucose. Patients with liver disease may have difficulty liberating glycogen or carrying out gluconeogenesis. Cachectic patients are unable to meet increased energy needs.	Monitor vital signs. Identify at-risk patients, i.e. those with cardiovascular, pulmonary, and metabolic disease. Monitor blood gas values of and administer oxygen to appropriate patients. Monitor blood glucose levels of diabetic patients. Be alert to patient's nutritional intake. Avoid additional stressors: Promote rest and comfort. Avoid disturbing conversation around the patient. Provide the patient with information he desires. Keep the patient comfortably warm. Alleviate the patient's pain. Maintain the patient's normal sleep pattern, to the extent possible. Avoid loud noise, and bright lights.

Increased blood supply to brain, heart, skeletal muscles	Selective vasoconstriction secondary to catecholamine secretion	Decreased urine output, increased specific gravity, pallor, diaphoresis, anorexia, nausea, abdominal distention	Decreased circulation to kidney causes: Renin release that leads to vasoconstriction. Elevated RBCs leads to greater blood viscosity. Lactic acidosis from decreased oxygen supply to nonessential tissues	Monitor vital signs and urine output. Monitor bowel sounds. Avoid additional stressors.
Increased blood clotting	Catecholamine secretion stimulates production of clotting factors.	Thrombosis, stasis	Increased blood viscosity	Encourage deep breathing, leg exercises, the use of antiembolism stockings, and slight elevation of the legs; avoid pressure on the backs of the legs, and encourage early ambulation. Avoid additional stressors.
Increased intravascular volume	Secretion of antidiuretic hormone and corticoids leads to retention of sodium, chloride, and water, and excretion of potassium.	Decreased urine output, weakness, hypotension, irregular pulse, EKG changes	Fluid overload. Potassium depletion	Monitor urine output and specific gravity, intake, daily weight, skin turgor, integrity of mucous membranes, pulse, blood pressure, laboratory data, level of consciousness.

(continued)

Table 1-3 (Continued)
The Physiological Effects of Stress and Nursing Interventions To Avoid Potential Complications

Effect	Pathophysiology	Symptoms	Possible Untoward Effects	Nursing Interventions
Increased intravascular volume (continued)				Monitor for signs and symptoms of hypokalemia: serum potassium level, decreased peristalsis, abdominal distention, hypotension, dysrhythmias, muscle weakness and EKG changes. Monitor for hyponatremia: abdominal cramps, muscular weakness, headache, nausea and vomiting. Avoid additional stressors.
Increased insensible fluid loss	Hypermetabolism increases respiratory rate; decreased peripheral perfusion leads to diaphoresis.	Decreased urinary output	Fluid loss	Monitor urine output and specific gravity, intake, daily weight, skin turgor, integrity of mucous membranes, pulse, blood pressure, laboratory data, level of consciousness. Avoid additional stressors.
Altered immune response	Secretion of glucocorticoids alters the immune response.	Signs and symptoms of infection Increased temperature, reddened wound or incision	Wound infection, atelectasis, pneumonia	Use sterile technique when changing dressings. Encourage deep breathing and coughing and early ambulation.

			Catheterize patient only if absolutely necessary. Monitor vital signs. Watch for signs and symptoms of wound infection. Avoid additional stressors.
Decreased gastrointestinal activity	Stimulation of sympathetic nervous system	Increased secretions of digestive tract; decreased peristalsis; decreased bowel sounds; anorexia, nausea, vomiting, abdominal distention	Vomiting, abdominal distention, and aspiration	Listen for bowel sounds, check for abdominal distention, position the patient to avoid aspiration. Check laboratory data for potassium level. Avoid additional stressors.
Increased excretion of potassium	Secretion of antidiuretic hormone and increased protein catabolism	Anorexia, vomiting, abdominal distention, decreased peristalsis, dysrhythmias, malaise, muscular weakness	Potassium depletion	Monitor for signs and symptoms of hypokalemia: serum potassium level, decreased peristalsis, abdominal distention, hypotension, dysrhythmias, muscle weakness, and EKG changes. Avoid additional stressors.

(Adapted from Stephenson CA: Stress in critically ill patients. Am J Nurs 77 (11): 1807, 1977 identifies nursing interventions that support the body's protective mechanisms and prevent the development of complications resulting from the stress response.

| Summary

The perception of physical or psychological stimuli as stressors initiates a generalized nonspecific response, the extent and severity of which is determined by the stressors. Knowledge of the physiological effects of stress enables the nurse to implement interventions throughout the perioperative period that support the protective mechanisms and prevent the development of complications.

Bibliography

Adashi EY, Rebar RW, Ehara Y, Naftolin F, Yen SSC: Impact of acute surgical stress on anterior pituitary function in female subjects. Am J Obstet Gynecol 138(6):609–614, November 15, 1980

Bullock BL: Physiologic effects of stress. In Bullock BL, Rosendahl PP (eds): Pathophysiology—Adaptations and Alterations in Function. Boston, Little, Brown & Co, 1984

Cassmeyer VL: Neuroendocrine integrating mechanisms. In Phipps WJ, Long BC, Woods NF (eds): Medical-Surgical Nursing, 2nd ed. St. Louis, CV Mosby, 1983

Farr L, Keene A, Samson D, Michael A: Alterations in circadian excretion of urinary variables and physiological indicators of stress following surgery. Nurs Res 33(3):140–146, May/June 1984

Genuth SM: The endocrine system. In Berne RM, Levy MN (eds): Physiology. St. Louis, CV Mosby, 1983

Guyton AC: Textbook of Medical Physiology, 7th ed. Philadelphia, WB Saunders, 1986

Halter JB, Pflug AE: Effects of anesthesia and surgical stress on insulin secretion in man. Metabolism (Suppl 1); 29(11):1124–1127, November 1980

Hamberger B, Jarnberg PO: Plasma catecholamines during surgical stress: Differences between neurolept and enflurane anaesthesia. Acta Anaesthesiol Scand 27 (4):307–310, August 1983

Harris JS: Stressors and stress in critical care. Crit Care Nurse 4(1): 84–97, January/February 1984

Henze R: Normal structure and function of the central and peripheral nervous system. In Bullock BL, Rosendahl PP (eds): Pathophysiology—Adaptations and Alterations in Function. Boston, Little, Brown & Co, 1984.

Hug Jr CC, Kaplan JA: Pharmacology–Cardiac drugs. In Kaplan J (ed): Cardiac Anesthesia. New York, Grune and Stratton, 1979

Johnson D: Physiology of stress. Crit Care Nurse 4(6):111–112, November/December 1984

LeMaitre GD, Finnegan JA: The Patient in Surgery: A Guide for Nurses, 4th ed. Philadelphia, WB Saunders, 1980

Long BC, Gowin CJ, Bushong ME: Surgical intervention. In Phipps WJ, Long BC, Woods NF (eds): Medical-Surgical Nursing, 2nd ed. St. Louis, CV Mosby, 1983

Marcinek MB: Stress in the surgical patient. Am J Nurs 77(11):1809–1811, November 1977

Miller Jr E: The renin-angiotensin system in anesthesia. In Brown Jr BR: Contemporary Anesthesia Practice, Vol. 3. Philadelphia, FA Davis, 1980

Moore RA, Smith RF, McQuay HJ, Bullingham RES: Sex and surgical stress. Anaesthesia 36(3):263–267, 1981

Oyama T: Influence of general anesthesia and surgical stress on endocrine function. Contemp Anesth Pract 3:173–184, 1980

Selye H: The Stress of Life, 2nd ed. New York, McGraw–Hill, 1978

Stephenson CA: Stress in critically ill patients. Am J Nurs 77(11):1806–1809, 1977

2 | Preoperative Patient Assessment

The first consideration in prevention is the careful and complete
evaluation of the patient.

—Anna L. Rogers, C. Lee Sturgeon, Jr.

The successful outcome of a patient's perioperative experience begins with the preoperative assessment. Surgery is a planned assault upon the body, and the preoperative assessment helps identify factors increasing the risk of that assault. The information gleaned from the assessment is used and added to by nurses caring for the patient in the pre-, intra-, and postoperative phases.

The Nursing History

Preoperative care begins when the nurse introduces herself to the patient upon his admission to the unit. Ideally, the nurse who is going to be working most closely with the patient admits him and interviews him. She orients him to the room, explaining the location of the light switch, bed control, bathroom, telephone, closet, and call light. She introduces him to his roommate and explains such unit routines as visiting hours and mealtimes. If the nurse is going to be his primary nurse, she explains what this means.

Obtaining the nursing history is an extremely important part of preoperative nursing care. While gathering valuable information, including the patient's understanding of his problem and how it is to be treated, the nurse begins to develop a therapeutic relationship with the patient and his family and to prepare them, emotionally, for surgery.

The data that the nurse gathers enable her to see the patient as the unique individual he is and to identify those factors that may increase the risk of surgery. A nursing admitting history, such as shown in Figure 2-1, provides a guide for conducting the interview and a means for documenting the data.

If the form is clear and written in nontechnical language, the patient may be able to complete it himself. The nurse explains that the information the patient provides will help the nursing staff meet his needs. She asks him to complete as much of the form as possible and explains that she will return in

---

SECTION I: (May be completed by NA or RN)

Date:_____   Mode of Admission: ☐ Cart   ☐ Wheelchair   ☐ Ambulatory

Time:_____   Accompanied by:_____   Relationship:_____

T.P.R._____   B/P_____   Wt._____   Ht._____

☐ Dentures   ☐ Partial   ☐ Braces   ☐ Caps/Bridge_____   ☐ Glasses   ☐ Contacts_____

Oriented to Unit: ☐ Yes   ☐ No   Signature:_____

- -

SECTION II: (Completed by RN)

Source of Information: ☐ Patient   ☐ Family   ☐ Old Chart   ☐ Other:_____

Drug Allergies: (Describe reaction)   ☐ NO KNOWN ALLERGIES

_____

_____

Food or Contact Allergies:_____

_____

YES   NO   YES   NO

☐   ☐   CBC/Coulter   ☐   ☐   ECG   Other:_____

☐   ☐   UA/Dipstick   ☐   ☐   Chest X-ray   Primary Physician:_____

Current Medications: ☐ Left at Home   ☐ Sent Home   ☐ Pharmacy Safekeeping   ☐ At Bedside

       ☐ NONE   (List medication, dose, time of last dose)

1._____   7._____

2._____   8._____

3._____   9._____

4._____   10._____

5._____   11._____

6._____   12._____

Chief Complaint/Reason for Hospitalization (includes history of present illness)

_____

_____

_____

_____

_____ R.N. Signature:_____

Figure 2-1. Nursing history form. (Courtesy Madison General Hospital, Madison, WI)

SECTION III: (May be completed by RN, patient or family member)

By what name do you wish to be addressed?_____ Occupation:_____

Marital status: M W S D Sep:_____ Pediatrics - Grade in School:_____

Do you have children? /_/Yes /_/No   Siblings:_____

Do you want visitors restricted? /_/Yes /_/No   Who may visit?_____

Do you desire clergy visitation? /_/Yes /_/No   What religion?_____

PREVIOUS HOSPITALIZATIONS: /_/None   Date of most recent hospitalization:_____

Date:	Reason:	Date:	Reason:

HISTORY OF ILLNESS:	PATIENT: Yes No	FAMILY: Yes No		PATIENT: Yes No	FAMILY: Yes No
Heart Disease	— —	— —	Kidney Disease	— —	— —
High Blood Pressure	— —	— —	Seizures	— —	— —
Diabetis	— —	— —	Neurological Disorder	— —	— —
Arthritis	— —	— —	Mental Illness	— —	— —
Lung Disease	— —	— —	Infections	— —	— —
Cancer	— —	— —	Injuries	— —	— —
Other: _____	— —	— —	Blood Transfusions	— —	— —

SECTION IV:

HEALTH PERCEPTION - HEALTH MANAGEMENT

How would you describe your general health? /_/Good /_/Fair /_/Poor

What medical treatment do you anticipate during this hospitalization?_____

Yes   No

___ ___ Do you smoke? Amount each day?_____
___ ___ Have a cough? _____
___ ___ Shortness of breath? _____
___ ___ Pain in chest? _____
___ ___ Other: _____
___ ___ Do you drink alcoholic beverages? Amount each day? _____
___ ___ Do you use recreational drugs? _____
___ ___ Do you take non-prescription drugs? _____
___ ___ Do you take prescription drugs regularly as prescribed? _____
___ ___ Do you feel you have a problem related to use of alcohol or drugs?_____
Comments:_____

NUTRITION - METABOLIC

___ ___ Do you follow a special diet? What type?_____
        How many meals do you eat each day?_____ Describe appetite: /_/Good /_/Fair /_/Poor
___ ___ Have you had a recent weight change? /_/Gain /_/Loss Amount:____ Normal Wt.:____
        Do you have any of the following problems?
___ ___ Abdominal Pain? Location:_____
___ ___ Constipation/Diarrhea_____
___ ___ Difficulty chewing or swallowing_____
___ ___ Nausea/Vomiting_____
___ ___ Bleeding or pain with bowel movement_____
___ ___ Pain with urination_____
___ ___ Problem with control of bladder or bowel_____
___ ___ Dark colored urine_____
___ ___ Frequent urination: /_/Day /_/Night_____
___ ___ Problems with your skin (sores, rashes, lumps, etc.)_____
___ ___ Swelling any place in your body (arms, legs, neck, abdomen, feet, etc.)_____
Comments:_____

Do you wear: /_/Dentures /_/Upper /_/Lower /_/Braces /_/Other_____
___ ___ Did you bring your dentures to the hospital?

ACTIVITY - EXERCISE

___ ___ Do you have any physical disabilities?_____
___ ___ Do you use a: /_/Cane /_/Walker /_/Wheelchair /_/Prosthesis /_/Other_____
___ ___ Do you exercise on a regular basis?_____
___ ___ Do you have pain in your joints, back, neck, arms, legs, etc.?_____

Figure 2-1. (continued)

SECTION IV (continued):

(Yes) (No)

Indicate level of independence in physical care:

	SELF	NEEDS ASSIST	UNABLE	Comments:_____
Feed				_____
Bathe				_____
Dress				_____
Walk				_____

SLEEP - REST

___ ___ Do you have problems sleeping?_____

_____

What are your usual hours of sleep?_____

Comments: _____

COGNITIVE - PERCEPTION

___ ___ Do you have difficulty hearing? Do you wear a hearing aide? /_/Right /_/Left
___ ___ Do you have problems with your vision? Do you wear: /_/Glasses /_/Contacts
___ ___ Did you bring: /_/Hearing Aide /_/Glasses /_/Contacts - to the hospital?

___ ___ Have you noted a recent change in your memory?_____
___ ___ Do you have headaches frequently?_____
___ ___ Are you dizzy or fall frequently?_____
___ ___ Have you had seizures or loss of consciousness?_____
___ ___ Do you have weakness of arms or legs?_____
___ ___ Do you have problems with speaking?_____

Comments:_____

_____

SEXUALITY - REPRODUCTIVE

___ ___ Any concerns or changes regarding your sexuality?_____
         Females: Last menstrual period_____
___ ___ Are you pregnant?_____
___ ___ Do you do self breast exam?_____
___ ___ Males: Do you do routine testicular exam?_____

Comments:_____

_____

SELF PERCEPTION - SELF CONCEPT

___ ___ Do you experience frequent changes of mood or behavior?_____
___ ___ Do you feel depressed? _____
___ ___ Are you often tense or upset?_____
___ ___ Do you have difficulty expressing your feelings to others?_____

Comments:_____

_____

ROLES - RELATIONSHIPS - VALUES - BELIEFS

         Who do you live with?_____
         Are there concerns/problems with this situation?_____
___ ___ Do you anticipate need for assistance at time of discharge?_____

___ ___ Have there been any recent changes in your life?_____

___ ___ Do you feel a need for more support from family or friends?_____
___ ___ Are there situations in your life that are affecting your illness?_____

___ ___ Are there religious or cultural practices that may interfere with hospitalization?

         Who do you want contacted in case of emergency?_____

         Name/Relationship_____ Phone No._____

         Anything else you would like to mention?_____

_____

_____

_____   _____
Patient/Family Signature   RN Signature

Figure 2-1. (continued)

15 or 20 minutes to discuss his answers. If the form is too complicated or too technical, or if the patient is too ill, the nurse completes the form herself. In either situation the patient interview is critical because it enables the nurse to see the patient as a person and not merely as data.

A surgical procedure, whether classified as major or minor (see the classification chart on page 28) is major to most patients and is always a stressor. The cost of this planned assault to the patient depends upon the surgical procedure itself and upon the patient's physical and emotional status. Knowing that a variety of factors can affect a patient's recovery, the nurse pays particular attention to the events of the patient's previous hospitalizations and surgeries, and assesses his nutritional status, fluid and electrolyte balance, general health, current medications, age, and emotional status.

| Previous Hospitalizations and Surgeries

Asking the patient to describe previous hospitalizations and surgeries can elicit invaluable information about the physiologic and psychologic aspects of these experiences. The nurse uses this information to plan and implement interventions that minimize the physiologic and psychologic stress of this hospitalization and surgery.

Malignant Hyperthermia

It is important to ask specifically about previous surgeries and experiences with anesthetic agents in order to identify clues suggesting malignant hyperthermia. Current literature suggests that one in 200 persons may be at risk for malignant hyperthermia. Typically these persons are healthy young adults.

Malignant hyperthermia is an inherited muscle disorder triggered by certain anesthetics, anesthesia adjuncts, and environmental factors such as stress. The pharmacologic agents most frequently implicated are inhalation anesthetics such as halothane and methoxyflurane, muscle relaxants such as succinylcholine, and amide-type local anesthetics such as lidocaine.

Most incidences of malignant hyperthermia occur the first time a person is anesthetized, and it becomes evident 10 to 20 minutes after induction. However, one third of cases may not occur until a second anesthesia. Similarly, malignant hyperthermia may not become clinically evident until the postoperative period.

Malignant hyperthermia involves an abnormal transport of calcium, resulting in increased intracellular calcium. Normally, when muscles contract, calcium is released from the sarcoplasmic reticulum (the calcium storing membrane of the muscle cell) and then, when muscles relax, the system takes up the calcium. However, in malignant hyperthermia the increased intracellular calcium causes generalized muscle contraction and fasiculations. Muscle oxygen consumption and lactate production increase. As intracellular mechanisms try to check the increasing calcium, the increasing aerobic and anaerobic metabolism causes metabolic and respiratory acidosis. The acidosis affects membrane permeability, and increasing muscle metabolism results in increases in lactate, carbon dioxide, energy, and heat. The patient's temperature

Classification of Surgery According to Degree of Risk

Classification	Contributing Factors	Examples
Major	Involves significant patient risk.	Radical neck dissection
	Long operating time.	Abdominal-perineal resection
	Significant blood loss.	Carotid endarterectomy
	Removal or handling of a vital organ.	
	Potential for postoperative complications.	
	Emergency procedure.	
Minor	Does not involve significant patient risk.	Excision of a sebaceous cyst on the scalp
	Brief operating time.	Removal of a wart
	Minimal blood loss.	Skin biopsy
	Few potential complications.	

may increase 1°C every five minutes. Although the patient's temperature is usually 39°C to 42°C, it may reach 44°C to 46°C.

Sympathetic nervous stimulation increases circulating catecholamines, which lead to tachycardia, dysrhythmias, hypotension, decreased cardiac output, and cardiac arrest. Other clinical manifestations associated with malignant hyperthermia include tachypnea, hyperventilation, and oliguria.

The mortality rate of malignant hyperthermia exceeds 50%. Therefore, preoperative identification of patients at risk is imperative. Assessment findings warranting further evaluation include:

>History of unexplained muscle cramps and/or weakness, accompanied by unexplained temperature elevation
>
>Presence of congenital musculoskeletal abnormalities such as club foot, hernia, strabismus, and ptosis
>
>Presence of round and bulky muscle groups
>
>Unexplained death of a family member during or shortly after surgery and associated with a febrile response
>
>Relative who had muscle rigidity associated with brown-colored urine and severe muscle aches upon awakening from anesthesia.

Nutritional Status

A patient's nutritional status is assessed preoperatively because it is directly related to intraoperative success and postoperative recovery. Malnutrition and nutritional deficiencies contribute to the increased morbidity and mortality of surgical patients. The various nutrients and their contributions to wound healing and operative success are summarized in Table 2-1.

Although the body's metabolic rate and need for nutrients increases during the perioperative period, its intake is usually less than normal. Healthy or marginally healthy patients tolerate this period of starvation and negative nitrogen balance, but malnourished patients do not. Therefore, when assessing the preoperative patient, the nurse is alert to factors predisposing to malnutrition such as reduced intake of food, reduced utilization of food, and increased energy needs. (See the chart on page 32.)

Malnutrition

Malnutrition is "a state of impaired functional ability, structural integrity, or development that occurs because of a discrepancy between the supply of essential nutrients and calories and the body's specific biological demand for them."[1] Surgical patients can demonstrate two types of malnutrition: protein-calorie or protein. Although the type depends upon the patient's prehospital nutritional state, estimates are that 50% of all hospitalized patients have protein-calorie malnutrition.[1,2,3,]

Protein is an essential component of cellular structure and is needed for survival. Two types of protein are found in the body — muscle and visceral. Muscle protein is used to perform muscle activity. Visceral protein is used to build and repair tissues and to fight infection and respond to surgical stressors.

Protein-calorie malnutrition or marasmus develops in the healthy surgical patient. Both protein and caloric intake are inadequate to meet the body's needs. Therefore, the body depletes its carbohydrate stores and mobilizes its body protein for energy. As a result, the patient rapidly loses muscle mass. Other signs and symptoms are brittle nails, weight loss, a history of anorexia, and dry, dull, sparse hair. Only in the late stages of protein-calorie malnutrition are visceral proteins depleted. At this time serum albumin and serum protein levels are decreased, and cell-mediated immunity may be impeded.

Protein malnutrition or kwashiorkor develops in chronically ill patients who have had an inadequate protein intake for a period of time. This inadequate intake can be due to the surgical treatment of a disease, such as a gastrectomy, or to an underlying medical condition such as chronic obstructive pulmonary disease, ulcerative colitis, or Crohn's disease. Regardless of the underlying cause, protein intake is inadequate to meet the body's daily requirements. But because the caloric intake is adequate, the patient does not lose weight rapidly. In fact, he may maintain his normal weight or even gain weight, depending upon caloric intake. However, if a significant protein deficit occurs, visceral protein is depleted. This protein malnutrition is evidenced by a decrease in lymphocytes, serum albumin, and transferrin levels.

Measures of Nutritional Status

Preoperative assessment of the patient's nutritional status is vital. It not only determines his current nutritional status, but also helps predict the conse-

Table 2-1
Nutrients Affecting Wound Healing

Nutrient	Specific Component	Contribution to Wound Healing
Proteins	Amino acids	Needed for neovascularization, lymphocyte formation, fibroblast proliferation, collagen synthesis, and wound remodelling.
		Required for certain cell-mediated responses including phagocytosis and intracellular killing of bacteria.
	Albumin	Prevents wound edema secondary to low serum oncotic pressure.
Carbohydrates	Glucose	Needed for energy requirement of leukocytes and fibroblasts to function in inhibiting activities of wound infection.
Fats	Essential unsaturated fatty acids	Serve as building blocks for prostaglandins that regulate cellular metabolism, inflammation, and circulation.
	a. Linoleic b. Linolenic c. Arachidonic	Are constituents of triglycerides and fatty acids contained in cellular and subcellular membranes.
Vitamins	Ascorbic acid	Hydroxylates proline and lysine in collagen synthesis.
		Enhances capillary formation and decreases capillary fragility.
		Is a necessary component of complement that functions in immune reactions and increases defenses to infection.
	B complex	Serve as cofactors of enzyme systems.
	Pyridoxine, pantothenic and folic acid	Required for antibody formation and white blood cell function.

	A	Enhances epithelialization of cell membranes.
		Enhances rate of collagen synthesis and cross-linking of newly formed collagen.
	D	Antagonizes the inhibitory effects of glucocorticoids on cell membranes.
		Necessary for absorption, transport, and metabolism of calcium.
		Indirectly affects phosphorus metabolism.
	E	No special role known; may be important if there is a fatty acid deficiency.
	K	Needed for synthesis of prothrombin and clotting factors VII, IX, and X.
		Required for synthesis of calcium-binding protein.
Minerals	Zinc	Stabilizes cell membranes.
		Needed for cell mitosis and cell proliferation in wound repair.
	Iron	Needed for hydroxylation of proline and lysine in collagen synthesis.
		Enhances bactericidal activity of leukocytes.
		Secondarily, deficiency may cause decrease in oxygen transport to wound.
	Copper	Is an integral part of the enzyme, lysyloxidase, that catalyzes formation of stable collagen crosslinks.

Developed from Levenson S, Seifter E.: Dysnutrition, wound healing, and resistance to infection. Clin Plast Surg 4(3):375 – 388, July, 1977
From Schumann D: Preoperative measures to promote wound healing. Nurs Clin North Am 14(4): 696, December, 1979

Factors Predisposing to Malnutrition

Reduced intake of food due to:

Faulty selection of foods

Poverty

Inability to swallow

Poorly fitting dentures

Unpalatable therapeutic diet

Lack of energy to prepare or eat foods

Unable to eat for 10 or more days

Long-term maintenance on I.V. dextrose solution

Anorexia

Reduced utilization of food due to:

Colitis

Pancreatitis

Alcoholism

Cancer

Diarrhea

Vomiting

Malabsorption

Increased energy needs due to:

Trauma

Wound drainage

Burns

Febrile disease

Cancer

Catabolic steroids

Stotts N: Nutritional assessment before surgery. AORN J 35(2):208, 1982

quences of inadequate intake for 10 days or more. The body's fat and protein stores reflect the patient's current nutritional status, while the patient's history provides clues to causes of malnutrition.

Physical examination provides objective data about the patient's nutritional state. To determine the degree of deficit, actual findings are compared to a standard. Malnutrition is mild if the physical measure meets 90% or more of the standard. It is moderate if the measure meets 60% to 90% of the standard and it is severe if it is 60% or less of the standard.

Three measures of nutritional status are anthropomorphic, biochemical, and immunologic. Of these measures those most closely associated with increased perioperative morbidity and mortality are biochemical and immunologic, specifically, abnormal serum albumin, abnormal serum transferrin, and delayed cutaneous hypersensitivity.

Anthropometric Standards

Numerous physical changes accompany malnutrition and multiple measures are used to identify it. Widely accepted physical measures of body mass or anthropometric standards include height, weight, triceps skinfold (TSF), midarm circumference (MAC), and midarm muscle circumference (MAMC).

Height and weight, which should be personally determined by the nurse, give a picture of the patient's anthropometric status. If the patient has recently lost or gained weight, the nurse should ascertain if the change was planned. Table 2-2 lists the ideal weight for men and women and also explains how to determine a patient's frame size. However, since the height–weight index is standard for the normal population, it may not accurately indicate the nutritional status of obese or edematous patients. Its application, therefore, is limited.

Triceps skinfold (TSF) adequately measures the body's fat mass, the body's major energy store. Since a pound of fat contains 3500 kcal of stored energy, only a major loss indicates a significant depletion.

The midarm muscle circumference (MAMC) accurately indicates the body's protein state. The MAMC is calculated from TSF and MAC. Table 2-3 lists the standards for anthropometric measurements.

Biochemical Measures

The two biochemical measures used most frequently to determine the status of the body's visceral protein are serum albumin and transferrin (iron-binding protein). Visceral protein is quickly lost during stress, and these biochemical measures indicate the severity of the loss.

Albumin reflects visceral protein because it is the major protein fraction produced by the liver. The liver metabolizes ingested proteins and creates protein fractions that contribute to both visceral and cellular protein functions. Serum albumin levels below 3.5 mg/dl indicate protein depletion.

Transferrin is an iron binding protein complex, the transport form of iron in the body. An adequate transferrin level is 200 mg/dl.

Immunologic Measures

The status of the cellular immune system reflects visceral protein. The total lymphocyte count and the test for recall skin-test antigens indicate the visceral protein compartment. Lymphocyte production requires protein and, there-

Table 2-2
Height & Weight Tables

How to Approximate Frame Size

Extend patient's arm and bend forearm upward at 90° angle. With fingers straight, turn inside of wrist toward body. Place your thumb and index finger on the prominent bones on either side of elbow. Measure space between thumb and forefinger against ruler or tape measure. Compare with measurements listed on chart which indicate elbow widths for medium framed men and women. Measurements lower than those listed indicate small frame. Higher measurements indicate a large frame.

Men (Height in 1" heels)	Elbow Breadth	Women (Height in 1" heels)	Elbow Breadth
5'2" – 5'3"	2½" – 2⅞"	4'10" – 4'11"	2¼" – 2½"
5'4" – 5'7"	2⅝" – 2⅞"	5'0" – 5'3"	2¼" – 2½"
5'8" – 5'11"	2¾" – 3"	5'4" – 5'7"	2⅜" – 2⅝"
6'0" – 6'3"	2¾" – 3⅛"	5'8" – 5'11"	2⅜" – 2⅝"
6'4"	2⅞" – 3¼"	6'0"	2½" – 2¾"

Ideal Weight*

Men Height	Small Frame	Medium Frame	Large Frame	Women Height	Small Frame	Medium Frame	Large Frame
5'2"	128–134	131–141	138–150	4'10"	102–111	109–121	118–131
5'3"	130–136	133–143	140–153	4'11"	103–113	111–123	120–134
5'4"	132–138	135–145	142–156	5'0"	104–115	113–126	122–137
5'5"	134–140	137–148	144–160	5'1"	106–118	115–129	125–140
5'6"	136–142	139–151	146–164	5'2"	108–121	118–132	128–143
5'7"	138–145	142–154	149–168	5'3"	111–124	121–135	131–147
5'8"	140–148	145–157	152–172	5'4"	114–127	124–138	134–151
5'9"	142–151	148–160	155–176	5'5"	117–130	127–141	137–155
5'10"	144–154	151–163	158–180	5'6"	120–133	130–144	140–159
5'11"	146–157	154–166	161–184	5'7"	123–136	133–147	143–163
6'0"	149–160	157–170	164–188	5'8"	126–139	136–150	146–167
6'1"	152–164	160–174	168–192	5'9"	129–142	139–153	149–170
6'2"	155–168	164–178	172–197	5'10"	132–145	142–156	152–173
6'3"	158–172	167–182	176–202	5'11"	135–148	145–159	155–176
6'4"	162–176	171–187	181–207	6'0"	138–151	148–162	158–179

*Weights at ages 25–59 based on lowest mortality. Source of basic data: 1979 Build Study, Society of Actuaries and Association of Life Insurance Medical Directors of America, 1980.
Reprinted with the permission of Metropolitan Life Insurance Companies © 1983.

Table 2-3
Standards for Anthropometric Measurements

Triceps skinfold (TSF)
Male   12.5 mm
Female   16.5 mm

Midarm circumference (MAC)
Male   29.3 mm
Female   28.5 mm

Midarm muscle circumference (MAMC)
Male   25.3 cm
Female   23.2 cm

Adapted from Blackburn G L et al: Manual for Nutritional Metabolic Assessment of the Hospitalized Patient. Boston, Nutritional Support Service of New England Deaconess Hospital, 1976.
Stotts N: Nutritional assessment before surgery. AORN J 35(2): 211, 1982

fore, the total lymphocyte count is an estimate of nutrition-related immuno-competence. Lymphocyte levels less than 20% of the total white blood cell count or an absolute level of less than 1500 may reflect protein malnutrition.

In the test for recall antigens, antigens such as PPD and Candida are injected intradermally. A patient with an intact immune system will develop a 5 mm induration around the injection site within 48 hours. The absence of such a response is diagnostic of malnutrition and is called anergy to recall antigens.

Obesity

Obesity can cause serious problems for the surgical patient. Although obesity is treated by weight loss if surgery is not emergent, the obese patient should not be placed on a calorie-restricted diet when admitted to the hospital. This will not lead to weight loss after discharge and may hinder recovery.

Obesity is defined as "that bodily state in which there is an excessive accumulation of fat in both the relative and absolute sense; that is, the percent of body weight present as fat is greater than normal, and the total body weight is abnormally high."[4] For the severely obese patient every pound of over-weight increases the surgical risk. An estimated 25 miles of blood vessels are needed to supply 30 pounds of excess fat! Blood volume, cardiac output, heart size, and pulmonary ventilation are increased accordingly. Obesity is associated with other factors such as hypertension, atherosclerotic cardiovascular disease, and diabetes mellitus, all of which may complicate the patient's perioperative course. In addition, the obese patient is at risk for aspiration and aspiration pneumonia because gastric emptying time is decreased and the acidity of gastric contents is increased.

Adipose tissue is relatively avascular. Its decreased number of blood vessels makes fewer white blood cells, fibrocytes, and nutrients available for wound healing. This decreased vascularity, together with the increased technical difficulty of surgery and prolonged operating time, increases the patient's risk of such wound complications as infection, dehiscence, and evisceration and hernia.

A larger than normal incision and more than normal retraction are required to extend the layers of fatty tissue in order to expose the surgical site. The retraction traumatizes the subcutaneous tissue. The larger incision and the excessive intra-abdominal fat make closing the incision more difficult and result in a larger dead space after suturing. This dead space and the trauma to the relatively avascular tissue from the retraction increase the risk of postoperative infection. Wound infection is a precursor of dehiscence and evisceration. In addition, the retraction may later result in incisional hernias.

Obesity decreases the efficiency of the respiratory muscles, and the excess body weight makes it difficult for the patient to cough, deep breathe, and move. Because the excessively thick chest wall and abdominal adiposity impede diaphragmatic descent, obese patients hypoventilate. Thus, pulmonary complications such as hypoxemia and atelectasis develop more frequently in the obese patient than in the nonobese patient. Although postoperative pneumonia probably is not more frequent in obese patients, special attention should be given to their pulmonary function. Early ambulation is encouraged, as is positioning these patients with the head elevated.

Fluid and Electrolyte Balance

Preoperative assessment of a patient's fluid and electrolyte balance provides valuable baseline data and helps identify patients at risk for fluid and electrolyte imbalances. This increased awareness helps avoid such intra- and postoperative problems as hypovolemia, hypotension, and cardiac dysrhythmias.

Some patients are admitted with fluid and electrolyte imbalances due to preexisting conditions, some of which are outlined on the opposite page. Others, however, develop fluid and electrolyte imbalances after being admitted. Just the stress of hospitalization can trigger the stress response which itself is associated with the retention of sodium and water and the excretion of potassium.

Body Water and Its Distribution

Total body water accounts for between 50% and 70% of body weight, depending upon age, the lean body mass : fat ratio, age, and sex. Adipose tissue contains minimal water. Muscle mass water content is 75%, while fat water content is 10%. Consequently, since women are less muscular than men, they have less body water than men. In both sexes the amount of total body water declines as age increases because adipose tissue replaces muscle.

Total body water is divided into two compartments: intracellular fluid (ICF) and extracellular fluid (ECF). Intracellular fluid is located inside the cells and accounts for about 55% of the total body water. Extracellular fluid is located outside the cell membranes and accounts for 35% of total body water.

Preexisting Conditions Predisposing to Fluid and Electrolyte Imbalances

Advanced age

Poor nutritional status

Prolonged fever

Draining fistulas

Intestinal obstruction

Burns

Chronic illnesses:

   Cirrhosis

   Diabetes mellitus

   Chronic obstructive lung disease

   Renal disorders

   Abnormal thyroid secretion

   Abnormal adrenal gland secretion

Anemia

Cardiac disease

Prolonged vomiting and/or diarrhea

Medications:

   Diuretics

   Steroids

   Laxatives

   Prolonged use of enemas

   Bowel preps for GI surgery

Fluid restrictions for laboratory and diagnostic tests

Extracellular fluid is further divided into plasma volume and interstitial fluid. Plasma volume and interstitial fluid account for 7.5% and 27.5% of total body water respectively. The remaining 10% is contained in bone and transcellular water.

Measures of Fluid Balance

Fluid balance depends on the following factors: fluid volume and osmotic pressure in the three main body compartments; fluid intake and output; renal function; the function of the endocrine system, and nutritional status. Fluid balance is assessed indirectly via such physical findings as daily weight, intake and output, urine specific gravity, vital signs, lung sounds, jugular venous pressure, skin turgor, and moistness of mucous membrane.

Plasma volume is estimated by central venous pressure and pulmonary artery pressure. Since these are pressures, they are functions of the plasma volume, the area within the blood vessels, and cardiac output. Therefore, factors other than changes in plasma volume, that is, constriction or dilation of blood vessels, can change these pressures.

Weight

When measured correctly, changes in daily weight over short periods of time are excellent indicators of fluid volume. For example, a weight loss of 2% of total body weight over 1 or 2 days indicates a mild fluid volume deficit. A loss of 5% of total body weight signifies a moderate deficit, and a loss of 8%, a severe deficit. Given the important data that daily weights can provide, it is imperative that the nurse personally weigh the patient when he is admitted. Subsequently, he should be weighed at the same time every day, on the same scale, with the same amount of linen, wearing the same clothing, before breakfast, and after voiding. Ideally, the same nurse weighs him.

An excess of fluid volume may manifest itself as edema. However, usually 5 to 10 pounds of excess fluid must be retained before edema becomes apparent. One liter of water equals 2½ pounds.

Intake and Output

An accurate record of total fluid intake and output can help detect discrepancies between gains and losses of body fluids. Twenty-four hour totals of all intake as well as all output provide invaluable information about the adequacy of fluid volume.

Just as it is important to note the volume of the fluids administered or lost, so it is important to be aware of the composition of those fluids. Table 2-4 lists the composition of various intravenous solutions, while Table 2-5 identifies the basic composition of gastrointestinal secretions.

The loss of large amounts of gastric and intestinal secretions results in hyponatremia and hypokalemia. However, while the loss of gastric secretions leads to metabolic alkalosis, the loss of intestinal secretions leads to metabolic acidosis. These imbalances are likely to occur when lost electrolytes are not adequately replaced.

Urine Specific Gravity

Urine specific gravity indicates the kidneys' ability to dilute and concentrate urine. Additionally, urine specific gravity can be used to assess the hydrational status of a patient with healthy kidneys. A highly concentrated urine indicates a water deficit, while dilute urine indicates either adequate hydration or possibly water excess. The normal range of urine specific gravity is from 1.003 to 1.030.

Vital Signs

Vital signs, particularly serial readings, rather than isolated values, provide valuable information not only about the adequacy of fluid volume, but also about electrolyte disturbances. Pulse, blood pressure, and temperature should be monitored.

Pulse rate indicates the adequacy of fluid volume and therefore should be checked not only for rate, but also for regularity, and volume. Tachycardia may indicate anxiety, pain, deficits in fluid volume and potassium, hypercarbia or hypoxemia. While a pounding pulse may indicate fluid volume excess, a weak, thready pulse may indicate a deficit in fluid volume and/or sodium.

Table 2-4
Composition of Intravenous Solutions

Solutions	Glucose (gm/l)	Na	Cl	HCO₃	K (mEq/l)	Ca	Mg	HPO₄	NH₄
Extracellular fluid	1000	140	102	27	4.2	5	3	3	0.3
5% dextrose and water	50								
10% dextrose and water	100								
0.9% sodium chloride (normal saline)		154	154						
0.45% sodium chloride (half-normal saline)		77	77						
0.21% sodium chloride (¼ saline)		34	34						
3% sodium chloride (hypertonic saline)		513	513						
Lactated Ringer's solution		130	109	28*	4	2.7			
0.9% ammonium chloride			168						168

*Present in solution as lactate but is metabolized to bicarbonate.

From Dudrick SJ et al (eds): Manual of Preoperative and Postoperative Care, 3rd ed, p 47. Philadelphia, WB Saunders, 1983

Table 2-5
Composition of Gastrointestinal Secretions

Type of Secretion	Volume (ml/24 hr)	Na (mEq/l)	K (mEq/l)	Cl (mEq/l)	HCO_3 (mEq/l)
Saliva	1000–1500	5–10	20–30	5–15	25–30
Stomach	1000–2000	60–90	10–15	100–130	
Pancreas	600–800	135–145	5–10	70–90	95–115
Bile	300–600	135–145	5–10	90–110	30–40
Small intestine	2000–3000	120–140	5–10	90–120	30–40

From Dudrick SJ et al (eds): Manual of Preoperative and Postoperative Care, 3rd ed, p 46. Philadelphia, WB Saunders, 1983

Postural hypotension is usually the first indication of a fluid volume deficit. For example, a drop in systolic pressure of more than 10 mm Hg from supine to standing or sitting usually indicates fluid volume deficit. However, a number of other factors can also cause hypotension. These include myocardial dysfunction, sodium deficit, severe potassium imbalances, a sudden shift of fluid from the plasma space to the interstitial space, and such medications as antihypertensives and diuretics. Conversely, hypertension can be caused by fluid volume excess, a shift of fluid from the interstitial space to the plasma space, hypercarbia, hypoxemia, anxiety, and pain.

Body temperature should be monitored because the increased metabolic rate that accompanies stress and temperature elevation leads to an increased loss of body water and electrolytes from the kidneys, lungs, and skin. A temperature of 39.4C (103F) increases the 24-hour fluid requirement by at least 1,000 ml. If correct amounts of the proper fluid and electrolyte solutions are not administered, fluid volume deficit and electrolyte imbalances can result.

A patient with a fluid volume deficit tends to have a subnormal temperature, as do the elderly. However, patients with serious hypernatremia, which is common in patients who are unable to perceive or respond to thirst, tend to have an elevated body temperature.

Lung Sounds

Lung sounds provide data regarding fluid status. For example, in fluid overload, bronchovesicular sounds may be heard in parts of the lung where vesicular sounds are normally heard. Rales that do not clear with coughing may be heard as congestion increases. Rales start in the bases and ascend as fluid overload progresses.

Jugular Venous Pressure

The external jugular veins are a valuable indicator of plasma volume. Normally, when a patient is supine the external jugular veins fill to the anterior border of the sternocleidomastoid muscle. Therefore, flat neck veins in a supine patient indicate a contracted plasma volume. A patient's inability to lie flat in order for the nurse to assess jugular venous pressure indicates elevated pressure.

Venous distentions extending higher than 2 cm above the sternal angle in a healthy person sitting at a 45° angle indicate elevated venous pressure. The elevated pressure may be due either to excess fluid volume or congestive heart failure.

Skin and Mucous Membranes

Skin elasticity or turgor and mucous membrane moisture indicate the status of a patient's fluid volume and electrolyte balance. For example, the skin of a patient with an adequate extracellular volume resumes its usual position after being pinched. However, the skin of a patient with inadequate extracellular volume remains raised for several seconds. This phenomenon is called *tenting*. In the elderly, tongue turgor more reliably indicates the adequacy of extracellular volume because the skin of an elderly person is less elastic. Skin turgor in all patients is best tested over the sternum or forehead.

While longitudinal furrows in the tongue are probably the most reliable sign of fluid volume deficit, dry, sticky oral mucous membranes indicate hypernatremia. Yet another generally reliable indicator of fluid deficit is the absence of moisture in the axilla and groin. A small amount of moisture should always be present in these areas and its absence indicates an extracellular deficit of at least 1500 ml.

Central Venous Pressure

Central venous pressure is an invasive means of measuring right-sided heart function. Since the catheter is introduced into the superior vena cava or right atrium, the central venous pressure provides information about the ability of that part of the heart to handle fluid volume. However, if a patient has chronic obstructive lung disease, right-sided congestive heart failure, or ventricular ischemia or infarction, the central venous pressure reading reflects changes due more to pathology than to fluid volume itself.

Pulmonary Artery Pressure

Pulmonary artery and pulmonary capillary wedge pressures are used to monitor left ventricular function indirectly. A flow-directed catheter, such as a Swan-Ganz, is used to obtain the necessary hemodynamic pressures. Changes in these pressures indicate early changes in left ventricular function and are of particular importance in patients with cardiac disease.

Electrolytes and Their Distribution

Just as fluid imbalance predisposes the patient to complications during and after surgery, so do electrolyte imbalances. The intracellular and extracellular compartments differ in electrolyte composition. The principal ions of the intracellular fluid are potassium, organic phosphate, and sulfate, while the principal ions of the extracellular fluid are sodium, chloride, and bicarbonate.

Measures of Electrolyte Balance

In the perioperative patient electrolytes of vital importance are potassium, sodium, and calcium. Tables 2-6 through 2-8 list the normal values for these electrolytes, their functions, signs and symptoms of imbalances, and preceding events. Signs and symptoms, as well as clinical significance, depend on whether the imbalances are acute or chronic.

Arterial Blood Gases

Arterial blood gas values are determined preoperatively when a patient has pulmonary problems or when pulmonary and/or cardiovascular surgery is scheduled. These values indicate adequacy of oxygenation and ventilation as well as disturbances in acid-base balance. The values of normal arterial blood gases are listed below:

pH	7.35 to 7.45
$PaCO_2$	35 to 45 mmHg
HCO_3^-	22 to 26 mEq/liter
PaO_2	75 to 100 mmHg
O_2 Saturation	94% to 100%

Table 2-9 lists selected causes and signs and symptoms of acid-base imbalances. Treatment is discussed in Chapter 8.

| General Health

The degree of risk that surgery poses to a patient is the sum of the factors inherent in three main elements: the existence of underlying diseases, the nature of the disease necessitating surgery, and the treatment. Preexisting medical conditions can increase a patient's risk for surgery. Therefore, the nursing and medical histories and physical examination, including laboratory and diagnostic tests, provide valuable information about the patient's ability to tolerate the stressors associated with surgery.

The function of various body systems is assessed, including the cardiovascular, pulmonary, renal, hepatic, endocrine, neurologic, immunologic, and hematologic systems. In addition, the patient's age, the medications he takes, and his coping strategies are considered.

Cardiovascular Function

The functional status of the cardiovascular system is a major indicator of how well a patient will tolerate anesthesia and surgery. Adequate cardiovascular function, including a heart that pumps efficiently, blood vessels that constrict effectively, and an adequate blood supply, decreases surgical risk. Assessment findings requiring further evaluation of cardiovascular function are:

(Continued on page 47)

Table 2-6
Functions of Potassium, Signs and Symptoms of Imbalances,
and Preceding Events

Normal Value:	3.5–5.0 mEq/L	
Functions*:	Transmission and conduction of nerve impulses	
	Contraction of skeletal and smooth muscles	
	Nerve conduction and contraction of the myocardium	
	Enzyme action for cellular energy production	
	Deposits glycogen in liver cells	
	Regulates osmolality of intracellular (cellular) fluids	
Imbalances:	Hyperkalemia	Hypokalemia
	Vague muscular weakness	Fatigue
	Nausea	Malaise
	Diarrhea	Anorexia
	Abdominal cramps	Nausea
	Bradycardia and cardiac arrest	Vomiting
	Oliguria or anuria	Abdominal distention
		Decreased peristalsis or silent ileus
		Muscular weakness
		Dizziness
		Dysrhythmia
Preceding Events:	Kidney failure	Excessive gastrointestinal losses
	Excessive administration of potassium	Use of potassium-wasting diuretics with inadequate replacement
	Adrenal insufficiency	Hypocalcemia
	Excessive use of potassium-conserving diuretics	Hyperaldosteronism
	Metabolic acidosis	Trauma, injury
		Metabolic alkalosis

*Adapted from Kee JL: Fluids and Electrolytes with Clinical Applications, 3rd ed, pp 91, 97. New York, John Wiley & Sons, 1982

Table 2-7
Functions of Sodium, Signs and Symptoms of Imbalances,
and Preceding Events

Normal Value:	135–145 mEq/L	
Functions*:	Transmission and conduction of nerve impulses	
	Largely responsible for the osmolality of vascular fluids	
	Doubling Na gives the approximate serum osmolality	
	Regulation of body fluids (sodium causes water retention)	
	Sodium pump action. Sodium shifts into cells as potassium shifts out — repeatedly — to maintain water balance and neuromuscular activity. When Na shifts into the cell, depolarization occurs (cell activity), and when Na shifts out and K shifts back into the cell, repolarization occurs.	
	Enzyme activity	
	Assists with the regulation of acid-base balance. Sodium combines readily with chloride (Cl) or bicarbonate (HCO_3) to promote acid-base balance.	
Imbalances:	Hypernatremia	Hyponatremia
	Dry, sticky mucous membranes	Anorexia
	Rough, dry tongue	Nausea
	Excitement	Vomiting
		Abdominal cramps
		Muscular weakness
		Convulsions
Preceding Events:	Decreased water intake	Long-term vomiting and diarrhea
	Increased urinary water losses when water intake is inadequate	Excessive administration of tap water enemas
		Administration of potent diuretics in combination with a low sodium diet

*Adapted from Kee JL: Fluids and Electrolytes with Clinical Applications, 3rd ed, pp 91, 97. New York, John Wiley & Sons, 1982

Table 2-8
Functions of Calcium, Signs and Symptoms of Imbalances,
and Preceding Events

Normal Value:	9–11 mg/dl	
Functions*:	Normal nerve and muscle activity. Calcium causes transmission of nerve impulses and contraction of skeletal muscles.	
	Contraction of heart muscle	
	Maintenance of normal cellular permeability	
	Increased calcium decreases cellular permeability and decreased calcium increases cellular permeability	
	Coagulation of blood. Calcium promotes blood clotting by converting prothrombin into thrombin.	
	Formation of bone and teeth. Calcium and phosphorus make bones and teeth strong and durable.	
Imbalances:	Hypercalcemia	Hypocalcemia
	Lethargy	Twitching around mouth
	Constipation	Tingling and numbness of fingers
	Anorexia, nausea, and vomiting	Hyperreflexia
	Decreased attention span	Muscle cramps and weakness
	Muscle weakness	Trousseau's sign
		Chvostek's sign
		Tetany
		Convulsions
Preceding Events:	Hyperparathyroidism	Inadequate protein intake
	Multiple fractures and	Extensive infections
	Multiple myeloma	Hypoparathyroidism
		Diarrhea
		Overuse of antacids and laxatives
		Renal failure

*Adapted from Kee JL: Fluids and Electrolytes with Clinical Applications, 3rd ed, pp 91, 97. New York, John Wiley & Sons, 1982

Table 2-9
Selected Causes and Signs and Symptoms of Acid-Base Imbalances

	Signs and Symptoms	Causes

Respiratory Acidosis	Acute:
	    Increased pulse and respiratory rate
	    Increased blood pressure
	    Feeling of fullness in the head
	    Mental confusion
	    Arterial blood gases:
	      pH$<$7.35
	      $PaCO_2>$45 mm Hg
	      HCO_3^- normal
	      $PaO_2<$75mm Hg
	Chronic:
	    Weakness
	    Dull headache
	    Arterial blood gases:
	      pH$<$7.35 or within lower normal if compensation has occurred
	      $PaCO_2>$45mm Hg
		Central nervous system depression
		Pulmonary dysfunctions:
		    Emphysema, bronchiectasis, pneumonia

Respiratory Alkalosis	Rapid, shallow breathing
	Inability to concentrate
	Circumoral paresthesia
	Arterial blood gases:
	    pH$>$7.45
	    $PaCO_2<$35mm Hg
	    HCO_3^- normal
		Hyperventilation due to anxiety, hysteria
		Gram-negative bacteremia

Metabolic Acidosis	Headache
	Confusion
	Drowsiness
	Increased respiratory rate and depth
	Nausea and vomiting
	Peripheral vasodilation
	Arterial blood gases:
	    pH$<$7.35
	    $PaCO_2<$35mm Hg
	    $HCO_3^-<$22mEq/L
		Uncontrolled diabetes mellitus
		Severe diarrhea
		Starvation
		Kidney failure
		Severe infections

Table 2-9 (Continued)
Selected Causes and Signs and Symptoms of Acid-Base Imbalances

	Signs and Symptoms	Causes
Metabolic Alkalosis	Irritability	Excessive intake of gastric acid neutralizers
	Dizziness	
	Tingling of fingers and toes	Vomiting
	Circumoral paresthesia	Hypokalemia
	Tetany	
	Arterial blood gases:	
	pH>7.45	
	PaCO$_2$>45mm Hg	
	HCO$_3^-$>25 mm Hg	

Enlarged heart
Evidence of cardiac failure:
    Dyspnea on exertion
    Increased venous pressure
    Enlarged and tender liver
    Edema
    Ascites
Hypertension
Significant valvular heart disease
Dysrhythmias
Angina pectoris
History of myocardial infarction
Peripheral vascular disease
Venous disease

Patients with cardiac disease are at greater risk for surgery than are noncardiac patients. However, the degree of risk depends on the cardiac condition and compensatory mechanisms. While minor or well-controlled heart conditions increase operative risk only minimally, other conditions contraindicate elective surgery. For example, moderate hypertension, with a diastolic pressure less than 110 mm Hg, does not contraindicate surgery. Similarly, neither chronic atrial fibrillation with a well-controlled ventricular rate nor an asymptomatic isolated right or left bundle branch block increases the risk of surgery.

Uncomplicated chronic hypertension without any evidence of coronary heart disease and mitral valve insufficiency increase operative risk only slightly. Likewise, mild cardiac failure controlled with digitalis and diuretics and not exacerbated by normal exercise increases surgical risk only slightly.

Cardiac conditions that are relative contraindications for elective surgery include recent angina pectoris, a crescendo change in the pattern of angina pectoris in recent weeks or months, unstable angina, severe aortic stenosis, high atrioventricular block (with symptoms like syncope), untreated cardiac failure, severe uncontrolled hypertension, and a myocardial infarction within the past 6 months. In the latter case elective surgery should be postponed for 6 months, if possible.

Pulmonary Function

The most common perioperative complications involve the pulmonary system. Respiratory conditions, including infections and chronic diseases, affect the patient's degree of surgical risk. Additionally, allergic conditions such as asthma and hay fever affect the choice of anesthetic agents. The presence of factors listed below signifies the need for additional evaluation of pulmonary function.

> History of smoking
> Inadequate nutritional status
> Obesity
> Advanced age
> Cough with expectoration of copious and/or purulent mucus
> Exertional dyspnea
> History of pulmonary disease
> History of heart failure
> Recent upper respiratory infection

Chronic obstructive pulmonary diseases (COPD) such as asthma, bronchitis, emphysema, and bronchiectasis increase the incidence of postoperative pulmonary complications. Chronic bronchitis and emphysema compromise the patient's ability to cough and exchange oxygen and carbon dioxide. Patients with severe COPD are in a state of compensated respiratory acidosis. Carbon dioxide is retained over a prolonged period, which causes compensatory renal retention of bicarbonate. This compensatory mechanism maintains the 1 to 20 ratio of carbonic acid ($CO_2 + H_2O$) and base bicarbonate. The extent of the COPD determines the severity of respiratory complications. However, perioperative factors that cause hypoventilation such as pain, narcotics, anesthetic agents, and immobility, exacerbate the complications. Unless adequate precautions are taken, the factors that cause hypoventilation can cause severe uncompensated respiratory acidosis.

Patients with lung disease who are scheduled for elective upper thoracic or abdominal surgery benefit from preoperative preparation. Although tailored to the patient's needs, the preparation always includes cessation of smoking for a minimum of one week. It may also involve the administration of antibiotics (for purulent sputum) and bronchodilators, and physical therapy to help remove excess sputum. By decreasing the incidence and severity of postoperative respiratory complications, this preoperative preparation also decreases the length of the patient's hospitalization.

Smoking adversely affects pulmonary function and increases the patient's risk of surgery. Smoking decreases the amount of functional hemoglobin available. Ten to fifteen percent of the hemoglobin may be in the form of carbonmonoxyhemoglobin (HbCO) and unavailable to transport oxygen.

Therefore, oxygen delivery to tissues may be impaired. In addition, because smoking reduces the formation of 2,3-diphosphoglycerate (2,3-DPG), the amount of oxygen unloaded at the tissues decreases. Smoking and chronic bronchitis also make airways more reactive, increasing the risk of airway obstruction. Secretions increase, gas exchange is impaired, and lung volumes are altered.

Renal Function

Kidney function is routinely assessed preoperatively because these bean-shaped organs play important roles in regulating acid-base and fluid balance, in excreting drugs and their metabolites, and in compensating for the stress of surgery. Although some renal conditions do not increase a patient's surgical risk, others do. If renal function is compromised, the stress associated with surgery can precipitate renal failure. Therefore, the presence of those findings listed below necessitates more extensive evaluation.

> Urinary frequency
> Difficulty in voiding
> Burning on urination
> Nocturia
> Polyuria or oliguria
> Periorbital edema
> Ankle edema
> Hypertension
> History of kidney disease
> Hematuria
> Proteinuria
> Hypoalbuminemia
> Elevated blood urea nitrogen and serum creatinine
> Electrolyte abnormalities

Chronic renal disease does not usually contraindicate surgery because of new management techniques. However, in patients with chronic renal failure, the ability of the kidneys to respond to stressors of the perioperative period is compromised. As renal function decreases, the remaining function is used to maintain the homeostasis of the extracellular fluid. Because minimal function is available to deal with the acute stressors of the perioperative period, the incidence of such perioperative complications as postoperative acute renal failure increases.

Pyelonephritis, glomerulonephritis, diabetes mellitus, and lupus also increase the risk of perioperative complications. This increase is due to the renal insufficiency associated with these diseases.

Liver Function

Acute and chronic liver diseases are important underlying disorders in surgical patients. However, the degree of risk that surgery poses is related to the severity of the disease. Assessment findings requiring further investigation are:

> Abnormal liver function tests

> History of alcoholism
> History of jaundice
> Ascites
> Hepatosplenomegaly
> Encephalopathy
> Poor nutritional state
> Prolonged prothrombin time
> Platelet deficiency
> Elevated blood urea nitrogen
> Decreased serum albumin
> Hyponatremia
> Hypokalemia
> Metabolic alkalosis

The liver performs a wide variety of important physiologic functions. It metabolizes proteins, carbohydrates, and fats, performs phagocytosis, biotransforms pharmacologic agents, synthesizes and excretes bile, and synthesizes the majority of the plasma proteins needed for blood coagulation. Since the liver biotransforms many drugs used in anesthesia, hepatic disease that affects their disposition potentially increases their toxicity and duration of action. In addition, liver disease is related to poor wound healing and an increased infection rate.

Endocrine Function

Since hormonal changes are associated with the stress response, diseases affected by these hormonal changes can adversely affect the patient's response to surgery. For example, changes in glucocorticoid activity and potassium levels can affect the body's use of insulin. In the diabetic patient the elevated blood glucose levels associated with the stress response can rapidly lead to diabetic ketoacidosis or hyperglycemic, hyperosmolar, nonketotic coma. Hyperglycemia results in fluid and electrolyte imbalances, and fluid loss or retention can further compromise kidneys already affected by diabetic nephropathy. In addition, diabetes mellitus predisposes to infection and impedes wound healing. Therefore, the disease should be well controlled throughout the patient's perioperative experience.

Adrenal gland function must be considered preoperatively because a patient's ability to tolerate perioperative stressors depends partly upon the ability of the adrenals to produce glucocorticoids. Normally the adrenal cortex secretes 15 mg to 25 mg of cortisol daily. But during stress such as surgery the adrenal gland can secrete 250 mg to 300 mg daily.

Adrenocortical insufficiency may or may not be known preoperatively. For example, insufficiency may be quiescent until the stress of surgery supervenes. Or adrenocortical insufficiency may be known preoperatively as in the patient with Addison's disease.

The most common cause of known adrenal suppression is the administration of exogenous glucocorticoids. This can result in adrenal atrophy, and the degree of resulting adrenocortical insufficiency depends on the dosage and duration of therapy. Sudden withdrawal of the medication preoperatively after intensive or prolonged therapy can lead to hyponatremia, severe hypotension with cardiovascular collapse, dizziness, fainting, fatigue, weakness, nausea, and hypoglycemia. Therefore, the nurse asks a patient about his use of steroids for more than two weeks during the past 6 to 12 months. If the patient has been taking steroids, his adrenal function may be checked by the infusion of ACTH. If the test results indicate decreased adrenocortical response, steroids are given preoperatively as well as intra- and postoperatively.

Just as adrenal insufficiency increases a patient's surgical risk, so does an increased level of adrenocortical hormones due to pituitary or adrenocortical disease. Excessive levels are associated with fluid and electrolyte imbalances, impaired wound healing, and increased susceptibility to infection.

Neurologic Function

Several neurologic conditions increase surgical risk. These include uncontrolled epilepsy and severe Parkinson's disease. Significant neurological findings in preoperative patients that warrant investigation include severe headaches, frequent dizziness, lightheadedness, tinnitus, unsteady gait, unequal pupils, and a history of convulsions.

Immunologic Function

Allergic reactions can be fatal. Therefore, the nurse asks the patient if he is allergic to any foods, environmental agents, or medications, and if he has ever had an allergic reaction, including a reaction to a blood transfusion. If he has, the nurse asks him to describe the "allergic reaction" in detail. When did the reaction occur? How long did it last? How did the patient feel during the reaction? What stopped the reaction?

Obtaining a history of the reaction is important because, to some patients, an allergic reaction is anaphylactic shock, while to others it is a few red bumps that itch. Even more commonly, patients term side-effects or an idiosyncratic drug reaction as an "allergy."

Hematologic Function

The adequacy of hematologic function can affect a patient's surgical risk and therefore is assessed preoperatively. Assessment findings requiring additional evaluation are:

> History of excessive or easy bruising
> History of excessive bleeding after a tooth extraction
> History of nosebleeds
> The presence of hepatic or renal disease
> Prior use of aspirin, anticoagulants, or antiplatelet drugs
> Abnormal bleeding time
> Abnormal platelet count
> Abnormal PT or PTT

Missing or abnormal coagulation factors increase the risk of hemorrhage and shock. However, blood conditions such as moderate anemia and various congenital and acquired hemolytic anemias do not contraindicate surgery. Usually they do not even increase surgical risk as long as the patient's blood volume and hemoglobin levels are adequate.

Smoking and certain medications such as aspirin have deleterious effects on blood coagulation and increase the patient's risk of surgery. Platelet function is altered in patients who smoke. Platelet stickiness and aggregation increase, clot retraction time decreases, and tensile strength of the clot increases. If the patient has smoked a long time, he will have an increase not only in the number of platelets, but also in the number of "adhesive" platelets. This overproduction and overactivity result in hypercoaguability that can have serious consequences for the surgical patient. Aspirin, in single analgesic doses, prolongs bleeding time by inhibiting platelet aggregation. Irreversible, the effect persists for the life of the platelet (8 days).

Just as the status of red blood cells and clotting factors are assessed, so is the status of white blood cells. An inadequate supply of white blood cells impedes the body's response to infection.

Any infection can adversely affect a surgical patient's outcome. Some infections indicate that elective surgery should not be done; others contraindicate it. For example, a cold, pharyngitis, or tonsillitis are relative contraindications to elective surgery, while acute lower respiratory tract infections such as tracheitis, bronchitis, and pneumonia absolutely contraindicate it. Furthermore, if the patient has an infection and the surgical site is near the lymphatics that are draining the infected area, the possibility of a postoperative wound infection increases.

The presence of such existing symptoms as sneezing, sore throat, elevated temperature, skin lesions, or elevated white blood count should be reported to the surgeon. Similarly, signs and symptoms of urinary tract infection should be reported.

| **Medications and Substance Abuse**

Many persons take a variety of prescription and over-the-counter medications. As the information in Table 2-10 indicates, some of these medications can exert adverse effects during the patient's intra- and postoperative period.

The nurse must clarify with the patient's doctor the patient's need throughout the perioperative period for such medications as antihypertensive and cardiac drugs, and insulin. It is dangerous to assume that a patient's medications are to be omitted simply because the doctor does not order them. He may have forgotten to do so.

When asking the patient to recall medications that he takes, the nurse asks him to mention *all* medications, not only those prescribed by a doctor. Frequently patients forget to mention birth control pills and over-the-counter drugs such as aspirin and antihistamines. The nurse lists those medications

Table 2-10
Medications That Can Affect Anesthesia and Surgery

Medication	Effects during the Intraoperative Period
Alcohol	May be associated with increased tolerance for anesthetic drugs; acute intoxication decreases the need for opiates and anesthetics, however.
Antiarrhythmics	
Propanolol hydrochloride	May depress myocardial function, thus decreasing cardiac output and pulse rate and may induce bronchospasm.
Quinidine gluconate, procainamide hydrochloride, and lidocaine hydrochloride	May impair cardiac conduction, cause peripheral vasodilation, and potentiate local anesthetics.
Antibiotics	
Aminoglycosides (kanamycin, gentamicin, streptomycin, neomycin, tobramycin)	Depress neuromuscular transmission and may produce mild respiratory depression; may potentiate neuromuscular blockade when combined with a curariform muscle relaxant.
Anticoagulants	Increase bleeding and hemorrhage; usually should be discontinued or the dosage reduced before surgery and the medication strictly monitored with serial coagulation studies.
Anticonvulsants	
(Long-term use of phenobarbitol and phenytoin sodium)	May increase metabolism of anesthetic drugs.
Antidepressants (monoamine oxidase [MAO] inhibitors)	Increase hypotensive effects of anesthetics; may cause hypertensive crisis when given together with sympathomimetic drugs.
(tricyclic antidepressants)	Cause hypotension because tricyclic antidepressants block norepinephrine reuptake at adrenergic nerve endings; cause tachycardia, urinary retention, and increase intraocular pressure due to marked anticholinergic effects.

(continued)

Table 2-10 (Continued)
Medications That Can Affect Anesthesia and Surgery

Medication	Effects during the Intraoperative Period
Antihypertensives	Many inhibit synthesis and storage of norepinephrine in sympathetic nerve endings, therefore altering patient's response to autonomic stimulation and stress. May aggravate hypotension; dosage may be reduced or discontinued before surgery. Abrupt withdrawal of clonidine (Catapres®) is often associated with rebound hypertension that can be severe. Clonidine is only available orally, and if the patient cannot resume it postoperatively, I.V. treatment with nitroprusside, for example, may be necessary to control the blood pressure.
Aspirin	Decreases platelet aggregation and potentiates the effect of anticoagulants.
Barbiturates	May be associated with increased tolerance for anesthetic drugs.
Digitalis	Dosage usually maintained and carefully regulated during intra- and postoperative periods. Digitalis toxicity is additive with hypokalemia.
Diuretics (thiazides)	Promote electrolyte imbalance; cause a constricted intravascular space and make these patients functionally hypovolemic under anesthesia.
Insulin	Dosage carefully regulated during intra- and postoperative periods. Often decreased or omitted preoperatively since anesthesia masks signs and symptoms of hypoglycemia.
Opiates	May be associated with increased tolerance for anesthetic drugs, if opiates are used chronically; acute use decreases anesthetic requirements.
Oral Hypoglycemic Agents	Depending upon the patient's status and procedure to be performed, the drug may be discontinued and the patient started on insulin. Some have prolonged duration of action and hypoglycemia can be a problem postoperatively.
Steroids	Decrease neuroendocrine response. If steroids have been used to treat a chronic problem (even though discontinued one month or more preoperatively), the increased demand during surgery usually requires an increased dosage. Exerts an anti-inflammatory effect and may delay wound healing.
Tranquilizers (phenothiazine derivatives)	May enhance hypotensive effects of other drugs; potentiate effect of narcotics and barbiturates.

that the patient is currently taking and has taken during the 2 weeks before surgery. For those medications that the patient is currently taking, the following information is obtained: name; dosing schedule; length of time the medication has been taken; reason for which it is being taken; time of last dose, and disposition of medications brought to the hospital.

The nurse also asks the patient if he uses alcohol and/or recreational drugs. Alcoholism and drug addiction are serious and widespread problems that increase surgical risk. Rarely will the patient admit that he has a problem with alcohol or drugs and skillful interviewing is necessary to identify such problems.

Alcoholism is defined by a history of excessive intake and physical dependence. This is indicated by the development of tolerance and withdrawal, psychologic dependence, and alcohol-related illness. Organ damage, associated metabolic abnormalities, anesthetic difficulties, and the potential for delirium tremens increase surgical morbidity and mortality. Delirium tremens postoperatively increase the patient's basal metabolic rate. In addition, they also increase postoperative mortality by 50%. Therefore, the following parameters should be assessed preoperatively:

History of abuse: what, how much, and how often
Chest x-ray
Complete blood count
Prothrombin time
Liver function tests
EKG
Serum electrolytes

Chronic alcoholism diminishes the adrenocortical response to operative stress and anesthesia. Therefore, chronic alcoholics have a reduced tolerance to stress. Alcoholics also have a cross-tolerance to anesthetics and analgesics. In addition, they frequently experience withdrawal symptoms, and their defense mechanisms against bacterial infections are impaired. They may also have such conditions as cardiomyopathy, alcoholic hepatitis, cirrhosis, and electrolyte abnormalities. If present, these necessitate postponing surgery, and if at all possible, surgery is delayed until withdrawal is complete.

Anesthetic and surgical risk in the drug abuser depend on the complications of addiction. Often the complications are not related to the drug itself, but rather, to the use of unsterile needles and diluents. Surgical risk seems to be greater in persons addicted to parenteral substances than in those addicted to oral substances. Some of the medical complications of drug addiction include infections such as skin abscesses and endocarditis, pulmonary edema, renal failure, acute and chronic hepatitis, peripheral nerve injury, thrombophlebitis, and intestinal "pseudo-obstruction."

Although some experts recommend that drug addicts or those on methadone maintenance be withdrawn from drugs preoperatively, this is often impossible. Generally these patients can be safely maintained on narcotic substitutes in the perioperative period. Methadone is the drug of choice for patients addicted to narcotics, while phenobarbital is the drug of choice for those addicted to sedative-hypnotics. Factors to be assessed preoperatively in the patient with a history of drug abuse include:

> History of abuse: what, how much, and how often
> Chest x-ray
> Urinalysis
> Liver function tests
> Hepatitis B antigen
> Blood urea nitrogen
> Creatinine

Age

Aging is an individual experience. Not all individuals age in the same way. Table 2-11 lists the aspects of normal aging and their effect on the patient's perioperative experience. However, since not all of these changes are present in all older individuals, and since not all are present to the same extent in each individual, preoperative assessment of the elderly is imperative. Assessment data are extremely important because even the elderly adult in good health has a rather slim margin of physiological functional reserve. When the patient becomes ill or stressed, as during the perioperative period, this margin narrows, sometimes drastically.

Although there seems to be no clear association between aging and surgical risk, cardiovascular and pulmonary complications cause the majority of deaths in the elderly surgical patient. Therefore, these two systems should be carefully assessed preoperatively. Similarly, careful preoperative assessment of an elderly patient's neurologic status provides valuable baseline data for postoperative comparison. Altered mental status is a common postoperative complication in the elderly.

Psychological Stress and Coping

Surgery is a personal experience that causes psychological as well as physiological stress. Therefore, the nurse includes questions in the preoperative assessment about those factors influencing a patient's perception of surgery. This information is used to assess the patient's coping strategies because situations alone do not define stress.

Perception of the Procedure

A number of factors can affect a patient's perception of surgery. These include its site, type and extent, the reasons necessitating it, when it must be done, and previous experiences.

A patient may perceive surgery as threatening when it involves such vital organs as the brain, heart, lungs, and kidneys. Similarly, he may perceive it as threatening when it is to result in the removal of a "meaningful" organ or necessitate an undesirable change in life-style.

Table 2-11
The Physiologic Effects of Aging, Their Significance to Perioperative Patients, and Related Nursing Implications

System	Changes	Significance of Changes	Nursing Implications
Cardiovascular	The number of elastic fibers in the heart decreases, resulting in rigidity. The cardiac wall stiffens. The endocardium thickens. The valves of the heart become rigid.	Cardiac output decreases; heart rate decreases and contractility of heart muscles is reduced. Cardiac reserve decreases.	Monitor patient for hypoxemia, shock, and cardiac failure. Minimize the number of stressors. Administer oxygen as needed.
	In the arterial system, the concentration of collagen increases and individual fibers stiffen. The walls thicken, and calcium and cholesterol accumulate in the vascular walls.	Peripheral resistance increases and peripheral circulation decreases.	Monitor patient for signs and symptoms of thrombosis. Initiate measures for preventing venous thrombosis.
	Sympathetic and parasympathetic nervous supply to heart decreases.	Ability to increase cardiac output decreases.	Monitor patient for signs and symptoms of hypotension and shock. Decrease the number of stressors and protect from falls from orthostatic hypotension.
	Conduction of impulses may become blocked due to anatomic changes in conduction system and ischemia.	Interrupted conduction impulses causes dysrhythmias.	Monitor patient for signs and symptoms of cardiac dysrhythmias.
Respiratory	Cross-linkage in collagen and elastic fibers around alveolar sacs increases; air spaces dilate; the number and size of alveolar pores increase, and lung tissue becomes less elastic.	Vital capacity of lung decreases about 25%; total lung capacity decreases minimally. Forced expiratory volumes and maximum breathing capacity decrease. Residual volume and functional residual capacity increase.	Monitor patient's respiratory status for signs and symptoms of failure. Administer oxygen as needed. Encourage mobility, unless contraindicated.

(continued)

Table 2-11 (Continued)
The Physiologic Effects of Aging, Their Significance to Perioperative Patients, and Related Nursing Implications

System	Changes	Significance of Changes	Nursing Implications
Respiratory (continued)		Reduction in number of alveoli can result in decreased diffusion surface for oxygen and carbon dioxide.	
		Blood oxygen level decreases; cerebral oxygenation decreases.	Institute patient safety measures.
		Inadequate elimination of carbon dioxide, combined with deterioration in renal and hormonal function, leads to electrolyte imbalances.	Monitor patient for electrolyte imbalances.
	Costal cartilages calcify. Thoracic skeletal deformities occur, postural changes occur, and intervertebral disks of thoracic spine degenerate.	Rib mobility decreases; chest wall compliance decreases; anteroposterior diameter may increase and the exchange of air between lungs and environment decreases.	Encourage pulmonary hygiene to prevent pulmonary infections.
			Monitor patient for signs and symptoms of pulmonary infection.
	Muscle tone decreases as does sensitivity to stimuli.	Cough reflex diminishes.	Monitor patient for signs and symptoms of respiratory infection.
	Epithelium dries and atrophies.	Ciliary mechanism becomes less effective.	Monitor patient for signs and symptoms of respiratory infection.
Neurological	The number of neurons decreases and they are infiltrated by lipofuscin and fat.	Losses occur in sensory functions, i.e., tactile sense decreases and pain tolerance increases.	Protect patient from pressure sores and other skin and joint damage.
		Intellectual ability remains stable.	Talk with patient as an adult, not a child.

	The nerve fibers degenerate and decrease in number.	Reaction time slows due to decrease of conduction velocity of impulse through peripheral nerves.	Institute safety measures. Give patient time to respond.
Renal	Anatomical narrowing and loss of vessels occurs and vasoconstriction is persistent.	Renal blood flow decreases.	Monitor patient for signs and symptoms of shock. Anesthesia and surgery significantly depress renal blood flow and glomerular filtration rate. Renal blood flow may not return to normal for 5 hours after surgery.
	The amount of connective tissue between the apices of the pyramids of the kidney decreases; the number of functionally intact glomeruli diminishes.	Glomerular filtration decreases, effective plasma flow decreases, as does reabsorption time.	Monitor patient for side-effects of drugs since drug excretion is often reduced.
		The ability of the kidney to form ammonia is impaired.	Monitor patient's fluid and electrolyte balance.
	Gross anatomical change leads to retention and stasis of urine and loss of power to sterilize urine.	Bladder capacity decreases. The sensation of the need to void may be absent or occur only when the bladder is almost full to capacity. Urinary frequency occurs and the residual volume increases.	Monitor patient for signs and symptoms of urinary tract infection.
	The prostate enlarges.	Normal urinary flow is obstructed.	Monitor patient for signs and symptoms of urinary tract infection.
Gastrointestinal	Diminished taste buds, loss of teeth, and loss of the grinding surface of molars.	Poor appetite and inability to eat can lead to malnutrition.	Encourage intake of nutritious, appealing meals. Order soft or mechanical soft diet, as appropriate. Assist patient with meals. Monitor intake.

(continued)

Table 2-11 (Continued)
The Physiologic Effects of Aging, Their Significance to Perioperative Patients, and Related Nursing Implications

System	Changes	Significance of Changes	Nursing Implications
Gastrointestinal (continued)	Hydrochloric production decreases.	Pernicious anemia develops due to absence of intrinsic factor in gastric secretions.	Monitor patient for signs and symptoms of pernicious anemia, i.e., anorexia, soreness of the tongue, and fatigue.
	Gastric mobility decreases.	Constipation occurs.	Encourage increased activity, fluid intake, and administer sedatives and narcotics judiciously.
	Abdominal muscles lose elasticity.		Monitor patient's bowel movements.
	Blood flow to liver is reduced, decreasing drug detoxification.	Drug toxicity.	Be aware of effects of drugs in the elderly.
Musculoskeletal	Bone resorption increases.	Brittleness of bone and tendency to fractures increases.	Carefully position patient on operating room table.
	Muscle mass decreases.	Muscle strength, endurance, and agility decrease.	Move patient carefully and gently.
	Joints degenerate.	Joints become stiff.	Carefully position patient on operating room table.
			Move patient carefully and gently.
Integumentary	Epithelial cells thin, which leads to prominence of bony markings.	Risk of pressure sores increases.	Implement measures to prevent pressure sores.
	Mitosis slows. Increased vascular fragility causes reduced vascularity.	Wound healing is delayed.	Promote wound healing via adequate nutrition and wound care.

Subcutaneous fatty layers thin; collagen and elastic fibers regress, and epithelial layer shrinks.	Skin becomes dry and inelastic; patient's susceptibility to cold environmental temperatures increases.	Avoid drying agents such as soaps; use lotion and moisturizers. Implement measures to prevent pressure sores. Do not use skin turgor as an indicator of hydrational status and keep the patient comfortably warm.
Sweat glands decrease in number, which prevents patient from sweating freely.	Susceptibility to heat exhaustion increases.	Monitor patient's temperature.
Melanocytes decrease	Caucasians become ''more white.''	Do not confuse pallor with anemia.
Sensory System Cochlea undergoes degenerative changes. Eardrum thickens, decreasing sound transmission.	Hearing is diminished. Difficulty hearing high-pitched sounds, and gradual loss of hearing.	Speak clearly, slowly, and in a normal tone while standing in front of the patient. Shut out extraneous noise.
The elasticity of the lens decreases.	Eyesight is diminished.	Make sure patient has glasses. Focus high intensity light on the area to be seen. Prevent patient from falling and injury.
Pupil size decreases due to increasing rigidity of the iris.	The ability to see in dim light diminishes.	Increase lighting to minimize falls. Keep a night light on in bathroom and along hallway.

Categories of Surgery Based on Urgency

	Classification	When It Should Be Done	Examples
I.	Emergent	Immediately	Intestinal obstruction
			Severe hemorrhage
			Perforated ulcer
II.	Urgent or Imperative	Within 24–48 hours	Kidney stones
			Acute gallbladder infection
			A bleeding duodenal ulcer
III.	Planned or Required	Surgery is scheduled weeks or months in advance	Tonsillectomy
			Cataract removal
			Hip prosthesis
IV.	Elective	Delay or omission of surgery has no adverse effects	Scar revision
			Hernia repair
			Hemorrhoids that are not bleeding
V.	Optional	A simple intervention based on personal preference	Face lift
			Mammoplasty
			Lipectomy

Surgery can be diagnostic, curative, restorative, cosmetic, and palliative. The purpose of a surgical procedure, together with its urgency, as identified in the "categories of surgery" listed above, can color the patient's perception. For example, a patient's perception of an emergency appendectomy, done to cure a disease, is likely to differ from his perception of a planned radical neck dissection done to treat a malignancy.

Previous hospitalizations and surgery, either the patient's own or that of close friends and family members, also affect his perception of a current hospitalization and impending surgical experience. Previous experiences may cause the patient to perceive surgery either as positive or negative, and he frequently transfers these feelings to the current situation.

Psychological Coping

A patient focuses his coping activities on the environment, on himself, or on the environment and himself. Coping activities have two main functions: to alter a stressful person-environment relationship, and to regulate the person's emotions arising from that relationship.

There are four major modes of coping. They include information seeking, direct action, inhibition of action, and intrapsychic modes.

Information seeking provides the patient with data that enable him to change his situation. The information may make him feel more comfortable by giving him a feeling of control.

Direct action can be used to change oneself, the situation, or one's interaction with the situation. For example, the patient uses direct action to alter himself when he stops smoking or loses weight several weeks preoperatively.

Inhibition of action is a patient's tendency to take no action. This occurs when he is completely convinced either that there are no direct ways of preventing the potential harm, that is, surgery, or that any action is too costly to take.

Intrapsychic modes of coping are cognitive processes that control the patient's emotions by making him feel more comfortable. These include the patient telling himself that "everything will be all right" and diverting his attention through avoidance.

Even though the nurse may deem a patient's coping strategies ineffective, she must not take them away unless she can replace them. Ineffective coping strategies are better than none.

Emotional Support

A key role of the professional nurse in the preoperative period is to help the patient and his family cope with the psychological stressors of the perioperative period. This may be accomplished by creating a supportive and trusting relationship and by assessing the patient's emotional state and coping strategies.

Surgical patients are normally slightly anxious. Moderate anxiety is helpful because it enables patients to identify fears and concerns and to deal with them. This anxiety may stem from "common" fears. For example, patients may fear that they will not wake up from the anesthesia, that they will reveal secrets while anesthetized, that cancer will be found, or that they will be in pain. However, surgical patients may have fears and concerns that are unique to them and unrelated to the surgery.

By creating a supportive and trusting relationship and by listening to the patient, the nurse makes it easier for him and his family to share their concerns and fears. The information gleaned enables the nurse to identify the patient's concerns, to assess his normal coping strategies, and to help him deal effectively with the psychological stressors of the perioperative period. For example, the nurse may learn that a patient derives much support from his religion. This knowledge enables her to ask him if he would like his clergy to visit. Only by knowing the patient as the unique individual he is can the nurse help him and his family cope most effectively.

| **Nursing Diagnoses**

During the preoperative patient assessment the astutely observant nurse recognizes clues that alert her to patients at risk. Many nursing diagnoses can be identified from preoperative assessment data. However, the most common diagnoses are listed below. These enable the nurse to develop and institute appropriate interventions.

Nursing Diagnoses Identified from Preoperative Assessment Data

Potential for ineffective airway clearance related to ineffective cough reflex

Alteration in thought process in the elderly related to environmental changes

Alteration in nutrition: Less than body weight related to inability to ingest nutrients because of biological factors

Potential for injury: Confusion related to environmental changes

Anxiety related to: Possible surgical findings
        Potential alterations in body structure and function

Knowledge deficit related to: Effective techniques for deep breathing, coughing, turning, and getting out of bed

        Surgical procedure

        Events of the immediate pre- and postoperative phases

From Kim MJ, McFarland GK, McLane AM (eds): Pocket Guide to Nursing Diagnoses. St. Louis, CV Mosby, 1984

Each diagnostic statement has its own goal. However, the overall goal for care derived from the nursing diagnoses identified as a result of the preoperative assessment is twofold: to prevent potential problems and to treat actual problems.

Communication of assessment findings and nursing care plans to the physician, operating room staff, and postanesthesia recovery room staff promotes continuity of patient care and ensures an uneventful intra- and postoperative experience for the patient.

| **Evaluation**

Factors that increase a patient's risk of surgery are identified and plans that minimize the risks are developed and implemented.

| **Summary**

With her knowledge and skills, the nurse is integral to the successful outcome of a patient's operative procedure. By seeing the patient as the unique human being that he is and by identifying the physical and emotional factors that increase his risk of surgery, the nurse hastens his uneventful recovery.

References

1. Stotts N: Nutritional assessment before surgery. AORN J 35(2):207, 1982
2. Cerrato. PL: Is your patient *really* ready for surgery? RN 48(6):69, 1985
3. Hensle, TW: Nutritional support of the surgical patient. Urol Clin North Am 10(1):109, February 1983
4. White JH: An overview of obesity: Its significance to nursing. Nurs Clin North Am 17(2):192, June 1982.

Bibliography

Arieff AI: Renal disease and the surgical patient. In Way LW (ed): Current Surgical Diagnosis and Treatment, 6th ed. Los Altos, CA, Lange Medical Publications, 1983

Association of Operating Room Nurses, Inc.: AORN Standards and Recommended Practices for Perioperative Nursing. Denver, The Association of Operating Room Nurses, 1983

Baesl TJ, Buckley JJ: Preoperative assessment, preparation for operation, and routine postoperative care. Urol Clin North Am 10(1): 3–17, February 1983

Blackwood S: Back to basics — the preop exam. Am J Nurs 86(1): 39–44, 1986

Blake DR: Physical assessment of the aged: Differentiating normal and abnormal change. In Burnside IM (ed): Nursing and the Aged, 2nd ed. New York, McGraw-Hill, 1981

Brock AM: How do the aged cope with surgery? Today's OR Nurse 6(9): 16–25, 1984

Brown FH, Shiau YF, Richter GC: Anesthesia and surgery in the patient with liver disease. In Goldmann DR et al (eds): Medical Care of the Surgical Patient. Philadelphia, JB Lippincott, 1982

Bullock BL: Physiologic effects of stress. In Bullock BL, Rosendahl PP: Pathophysiology-Adaptations and Alterations in Function. Boston, Little, Brown & Co, 1984

Burggraf V, Donlon B: Assessing the elderly. Am J Nurs 85(9): 974–984, 1985

Buzby GP, Mullen JL: Nutrition and the surgical patient. In Goldmann DR et al (eds): Medical Care of the Surgical Patient. Philadelphia, JB Lippincott, 1982

Carey KW: Caring for Surgical Patients. Springhouse, PA, Intermed Communications, 1982

Carrick L: Considerations for the older surgical patient. Geriatric Nurs 3(1): 43–50, January/February, 1982

Cebul RD, Kussmaul WG: Preoperative pulmonary evaluation and preparation. In Goldmann DR et al (eds): Medical Care of the Surgical Patient. Philadelphia, JB Lippincott, 1982

Cerrato PL: Is your patient *really* ready for surgery? RN 48(6): 69–70, 1985

Collard AF: Physical changes of normal aging. In Howe J, Dickason EJ, Jones DA, Snider MJ (eds): The Handbook of Nursing. New York, John Wiley & Sons, 1984

Coyne JC, Aldwin C, Lazarus RS: Depression and coping in stressful episodes. J Abnorm Psychol 90(5): 439–447, 1981

Demling RH: Preoperative care. In Way LW (ed): Current Surgical Diagnosis and Treatment, 6th ed. Los Altos, CA, Lang Medical Publications, 1983

Felver L: Understanding the electrolyte maze. Am J Nurs 80(9): 1591–1595, 1980

Folk–Lighty M: Solving the puzzles of patients' fluid imbalance. Nurs 84 14(2): 34–41, 1984

Forsham PH: Endocrine disease and the surgical patient. In Way LW (ed): Current Surgical Diagnosis and Treatment, 6th ed. Los Altos, CA, Lang Medical Publications, 1983

Fraulini KE: Coping mechanisms and recovery from surgery. AORN J 37(6): 1198–1208, May 1983

French MM, Phillips KF: When seconds count: Treating malignant hyperthermia. RN 47(11): 26–31, 1984

Glass LB, Jenkins CA: The ups and downs of serum pH. Nurs 83 13(9): 34–41, 1983

Glenn F: Surgical principles for the aged patient. In Reichel W (ed): Clinical Aspects of Aging, 2nd ed. Baltimore, William & Wilkins, 1983

Gronert GA: Malignant hyperthermia. Anesthesiology 53(5): 395–413, November 1980

Gruendemann BJ, Meeker MH: Alexander's care of the patient. In Surgery, 7th ed. St. Louis, CV Mosby, 1983

Guadagni NP, Hamilton WK: Anesthesiology. In Way LW (ed): Current Surgical Diagnosis and Treatment, 6th ed. Los Altos, CA, Lange Medical Publications, 1983

Henderson ML: Altered presentations. Am J Nurs 85(10): 1104–1106, 1985

Hensle TW: Nutritional support of the surgical patient. Urol Clin North Am 10(1): 109–118, February 1983

Hickey RF: Respiratory disease and the surgical patient. In Way LW (ed): Current Surgical Diagnosis and Treatment, 6th ed. Los Altos, CA, Lange Medical Publications, 1983

Hill GL, Church J: Energy and protein requirements of general surgical patients requiring intravenous nutrition. Br J Surg 71(1): 1–9, 1984

Hirsch RA: An approach to assessing perioperative risk. In Goldmann DR et al (eds): Medical Care of the Surgical Patient. Philadelphia, JB Lippincott, 1982.

Horowitz RS, Morganroth J, Levy, WK: Evaluation and management of the surgical patient with coronary artery disease. In Goldmann DR et al (eds): Medical Care of the Surgical Patient. Philadelphia, JB Lippincott, 1982

Hudson MF: Drugs and the older adult. Nurs 84 14(8): 47–51, 1984

Hudson MF: Safeguard your elderly patient's health through accurate physical assessment. Nurs 83 13(11): 58–64, 1983

Johnson JC: Surgery in the elderly. In Goldmann DR et al (eds): Medical Care of the Surgical Patient. Philadelphia, JB Lippincott, 1982

Johnson JE, Dabs JM, Leventhal H: Psychological factors in the welfare of patients. Nurs Res Vol. 19: 18–29, January/February 1970

Julien R: Understanding Anesthesia. Menlo Park, CA, Addison–Wesley, 1984

Kanner AD, Coyne JC, Schaefer C, Lazarus RS: Comparison of two modes of stress measurement: Daily hassles and uplifts versus major life events. J Behav Med 4(1): 1–39, 1981

Kee JL: Fluids and Electrolytes with Clinical Applications, 3rd ed. New York, John Wiley & Sons, 1982

Kim MJ, McFarland GK, McLane AM (eds): Pocket Guide to Nursing Diagnoses. St. Louis, CV Mosby, 1984

Kneedler J, Dodge G: Perioperative Patient Care. Boston, Blackwell Scientific Publications, 1983

Lazarus RS: Emotion and adaptation: Conceptual and empirical relations. In Arnold WJ (ed): Nebraska Symposium on Motivation. Lincoln, NE, University of Nebraska Press, 1968

Lazarus RS: Psychological stress and coping in adaptation and illness. Int J Psychiatry Med 5(4): 321–333, 1974

Lazarus RS, Cohen JB, Folkman S, Kanner A, Schaefer C: Psychological stress and adaptation: Some unresolved issues. In Selye H (ed): Selye's Guide to Stress Research, Vol 1. New York, Van Nostrand Reinhold, 1980

Levy WK: Alcohol and drug abuse in the surgical patient. In Goldmann DR et al (eds): Medical Care of the Surgical Patient. Philadelphia, JB Lippincott, 1982

Linn BS, Linn MW, Jensen J: Surgical stress in the healthy elderly. J Am Geriatr Soc 31(9): 544–548, 1983

Long BC, Gowin CJ, Bushong ME: Surgical intervention. In Phipps WJ, Long BC, Woods NF (eds): Medical-Surgical Nursing, 2nd ed. St. Louis, CV Mosby, 1983

Marchildon MB: Malignant hyperthermia. Arch Surg 117: 349–351, March 1982

Mauldin BC: Ambulatory surgery. AORN J 39(5): 770–771, April 1984

McConnell E: How nursing care plans help you. NursingLife 2(1): 55–59, January/ February 1982

Meckes PR: Perioperative care of the elderly patient. Today's OR Nurse 6(9): 8–15, 1984

Metheny N: Preoperative fluid balance assessment. AORN J 33(1): 51–56, 1981

Metheny NM: Quick Reference to Fluid Balance. Philadelphia, JB Lippincott, 1984

Metheny NM, Snively Jr WD: Nurses' Handbook of Fluid Balance, 4th ed. Philadelphia, JB Lippincott, 1983

Murray TG: The surgical patient with chronic renal failure. In Goldmann DR et al (eds): Medical Care of the Surgical Patient. Philadelphia, JB Lippincott, 1982

Noble E: Malignant hyperthermia need not be lethal. The Canadian Nurse 76(8): 33–37, September 1980

Owen CA, Bowie EJW: Disorders of coagulation. Urol Clin North Am 10(1): 77–87, February 1983

Pastewski BM, Gerbino PP: Drug reactions and interactions in the surgical patient. In Goldmann DR et al (eds): Medical Care of the Surgical Patient. Philadelphia, JB Lippincott, 1982

Phelps RL: Endocrine crises in surgical patients. Section A: Diabetes mellitus. In Beal JM: Critical Care for Surgical Patients. New York, Macmillan, 1982

Phippen ML: Nursing assessment of preoperative anxiety. AORN J 31(6): 1019–1026, May 1980

Podjasek JH: Which postop patient faces the greatest respiratory risk? RN 48(9): 44–56, 1985

Reichgott MA: Hypertension in the perioperative patient. In Goldmann DR et al (eds): Medical Care of the Surgical Patient. Philadelphia, JB Lippincott, 1982

Roberts SL: Cardiopulmonary abnormalities in aging. In Burnside IM (ed): Nursing and the Aged, 2nd ed. New York, McGraw-Hill, 1981

Roberts SL: Renal abnormalities in aging. In Burnside IM (ed): Nursing and the Aged, 2nd ed. New York, McGraw-Hill, 1981.

Rogers AL, Sturgeon Jr CL: Malignant hyperthermia. AORN J 41(2): 369–374, 1985

Rosenberg H: Malignant hyperpyrexia. Am J Nurs 81(8): 1484–1486, 1981

Ross AD, Angaran DM: Colloids vs. crystalloids—A continuing controversy. Drug Intell Clin Pharm Vol. 18: 202–212, March 1984

Rossman I: Human aging changes. In Burnside IM (ed): Nursing and the Aged, 2nd ed. New York, McGraw–Hill, 1981

Schumann D: Preoperative measures to promote wound healing. Nurs Clin North Am 14(4): 683–699, December 1979

Selye H: The Stress of Life, 2nd ed. New York, McGraw–Hill, 1978

Shanck AH: Musculoskeletal problems in aging. In Burnside IM (ed): Nursing and the Aged, 2nd ed. New York, McGraw–Hill, 1981

Silverstein DK, Karliner JS: Perioperative cardiac care. Urol Clin North Am 10(1): 51–63, February 1983

Sokolow M: Cardiac disease and the surgical patient. In Way, LW (ed): Current Surgical Diagnosis and Treatment, 6th ed. Los Altos, CA, Lange Medical Publications, 1983

St. Haxholdt O, Johansson G: The alcoholic patient and surgical stress. The Association of Anaesthetists of Great Britain and Ireland 37(8): 797–801, 1982

Stotts N: Nutritional assessment before surgery. AORN J 35(2): 207–214, 1982

Street MF, Earles V: Aging. In Bullock BL, Rosendahl PP (eds): Pathophysiology—Adaptations and Alterations in Function. Boston, Little, Brown and Co, 1984

Stuhler-Schlag MK: Pre and postoperative fluids and electrolytes. Today's OR Nurse 4(7): 11–15, 66–67, September 1982

Teasley KM, Lysne J, Nuwer N, Shronts EP, Cerra FB: Nutrition and metabolic support of the surgical patient. Urol Clin North Am 10(1): 119–129, February 1983

Wallerstein RO: Hematologic disease and the surgical patient. In Way LW (ed): Current Surgical Diagnosis and Treatment, 6th ed. Los Altos, CA, Lange Medical Publications, 1983

White JH: An overview of obesity: Its significance to nursing. Nurs Clin North Am 17(2): 191–198, June 1982

Williams SV: Perioperative management of the overweight patient. In Goldmann, DR et al (eds): Medical Care of the Surgical Patient. Philadelphia, JB Lippincott, 1982

Wong J, Wong S: Surgical care of the aged. The Canadian Nurse 77(11): 30–33, December 1981

3 | Preoperative Preparation

An ounce of prevention is worth a pound of cure.

Just as patient assessment is an essential part of the preoperative phase, so also is patient preparation. The nurse helps prepare the patient emotionally and physiologically not only for the surgical procedure, but also for events of the intra- and postoperative periods.

When preparing the patient, the nurse implements interventions aimed at achieving the goals of those nursing diagnoses identified after assessing the patient (listed in Chapter 2). Additionally, she may acquire new information that necessitates revising the nursing diagnoses, goals, and plans.

| The Operative Permit

A patient must give the surgeon permission to operate. Before voluntarily signing an operative permit, the patient must know what the surgeon plans to do and the potential complications associated with the procedure. This authorized permission protects not only the patient, but also the surgeon. The operative permit protects the patient from procedures that he neither desires to have performed nor understands. Similarly, the permit protects the surgeon and hospital staff from legal action in which the patient or his family alleges that surgery was performed without either the patient's knowledge or permission. Special permits for specific operations, such as sterilization, disposal of amputated body parts, and autopsy, are required and provide additional safeguards for the patient, staff, and hospital.

The surgeon is ultimately responsible for obtaining the patient's signed consent and for clearly and concisely explaining the procedure to him. He uses words that the patient and his family understand and may use models or draw diagrams to illustrate the procedure. In addition, the surgeon informs the patient of inherent risks and possible complications associated with the procedure. The patient must sign the surgical consent *before* being given any preoperative medications.

Any patient undergoing surgery must sign his own consent form, unless he is unconscious, mentally incompetent, or a minor. In such cases, a responsible family member or legal guardian may give permission. However, if the minor is "emancipated," that is, either married or financially supporting himself, he may sign his own surgical consent. A surgeon may perform a lifesaving procedure without obtaining informed consent, but every attempt should be made to contact the patient's family either by telephone or telegram.

Although the surgeon is responsible for explaining the procedure and its inherent risks to the patient, the nurse assesses the patient's level of understanding and readiness to sign the permit. Should she determine that the patient does not understand what is to be done or is not ready to sign the permit, she notifies the surgeon.

Frequently the nurse is asked to "witness" the patient's signature. That is, the surgeon has explained the procedure and its potential hazards, but asks the nurse to "get the permit signed." If the nurse obtains the patient's signature, she asks him if he believes that he understands what the physician has told him about the procedure and the risks involved. If the patient says "yes" and signs the permit, the nurse witnesses his signature. In addition, she documents in the nurse's notes that the patient stated that he believed he understood the physician's explanation. The surgical consent form is a permanent part of the patient's chart and usually is valid only for a certain number of days.

If the patient does not understand what the physician told him or if he wants more information, the nurse can answer questions within her level of knowledge. However, if she does not answer the questions or if the patient does not understand, the nurse does not have the patient sign the permit. She notifies the physician of the patient's need for additional information and documents her observations and actions in the chart.

Preoperative Patient Education

The purpose of preoperative instruction is to decrease the severity of the stress response and to minimize the occurrence of intra- and postoperative complications. Studies have shown that the well-prepared surgical patient has less difficulty undergoing anesthesia and has a shorter, less complicated postoperative hospital stay than does the unprepared patient.[1,2,3] Studies also support the benefits of structured versus unstructured preoperative teaching for adults with lower and upper abdominal surgery.[4]

Preoperative teaching can take a number of forms: individual, group, or individual *and* group. The form that best meets the patient's needs depends upon his age and psychosocial characteristics, including cognitive, emotional, body image development, and developmental tasks. Table 3-1 lists these characteristics for the young, middle aged, and elderly adult. Preoperative teaching, regardless of its form, must be tailored to meet the needs of the patient. Guidelines in Chapter 9 explain factors to be considered in developing a teaching-learning plan.

Most patients and their families want to know what to expect during the perioperative period. Seventy to ninety percent of surgical patients admit they have fears about anesthesia, surgery, or anesthesia and surgery.[5] But before providing ANY information, the nurse determines just what the patient and his family already know and what information they may want.

Just as preoperative instruction itself is important, so is the kind of information that the patient receives. Study results indicate that the kind of information a patient receives affects his degree of distress. Sensory information, together with procedural information, helps decrease a patient's distress. Sensory information describes the sights, sounds, feelings, odors, tastes, and temperature that he can expect. Procedural information, on the other hand, gives the patient facts about the procedure such as where it will take place, who will perform it, and how he will be positioned. Therefore, preoperatively, the nurse not only tells the patient what will happen intra- and postoperatively, but also describes sensations he may experience.[1,2,3]

A preoperative teaching guide, as illustrated in Figure 3-1, provides the nurse with an outline and a means of documenting the teaching and the patient's response to it. Because the guide is a permanent part of the patient's record, it facilitates communication and enables the nurse in the surgical reception area to reinforce teaching and to allay the patient's anxieties.

| Preoperative Instruction

The most frequent causes of death and morbidity in patients following anesthesia are pulmonary complications such as atelectasis, pneumonia, acute respiratory failure, and pulmonary emboli. Similarly, pain is a common sequela of surgery and its relief of concern to patients. Therefore, preoperatively, the nurse teaches the patient how and why to use an incentive spirometer, and how to deep breathe, sigh, yawn, cough, turn from side to side, exercise his legs, and get out of bed. Additionally, she explains the measures that will be used to manage his pain after surgery.

Voluntary Sustained Maximal Inspiration

Voluntary sustained maximal inspiration (SMI), defined as sustained alveolar inflation to maximal lung capacity, is extremely useful in preventing postoperative pulmonary complications such as atelectasis. Alveolar inflation to lung capacity is produced by high negative transpulmonary pressures. Transpulmonary pressure is the difference between positive alveolar pressure and negative

Table 3-1
Psychosocial Characteristics of the Healthy Individual

Age Group	Cognitive Development	Emotional Development	Body Image Development	Developmental Tasks
Young Adult (20 to 40 Years)	Thinking and learning are problem-centered Thinks at an abstract level and compares experiences with previous memories, knowledge, and experience Learns formally and informally by emphasizing principles and concepts	Sexuality is a powerful factor Appearance is highest priority Erikson's task: intimacy vs. self-absorption or self-isolation	Body image is flexible and may not reflect actual body structure	Establishes independence Establishes intimate bond with another
Middle-Aged Adult (40 to 65 Years)	Goal oriented Decreased memory functioning Retains less from oral information Problem-centered thinking	Self-assessment period Masters his environment Values age and life experiences Erikson's task: generativity vs. self-absorption and stagnation	Changes accepted as part of maturity Reinforces positive self-concept	Develops new satisfaction as a mate Balances work with other roles
Elderly Adult (Over 65 Years)	May decrease due to physiologic deterioration	Sense of wisdom, knowledge, and self-reliance, of being able to cope with whatever comes Erikson's task: integrity vs. despair	Integrates continuing physiologic changes May see body as less dependable	Recognizes the positive experience of aging Maintaining self-worth, pride and usefulness

Adapted from Am J Nurs 1985 Nursing Boards Review, pp 152–154

Discuss the following with your patient and his family.
Indicate date and your signature after completion.

DATE TIME INITIAL

I. Pre-Operative Period

   A. Food and fluid restricted NPO sign means nothing by mouth.

   B. Sleeping pill to insure rest.

   C. Shower/tub bath and prep before surgery.

   D. Pre-operative medication ("hypo") one hour before surgery.
     . Not induce sleep but aid in relaxation.
     . May experience dry mouth/drowsiness.
     . Remain in bed, quiet after.

   E. Transported to and from O.R. accompanied by O.R. staff.

   F. Information for the family.
     . May visit relative morning of surgery before going to Operating Room.
     . If operation scheduled for 8 A.M., leave unit at 7:15 A.M.
     . May wait in waiting room (4 Center) or in patient's room.
     . Inform unit secretary if the family leaves the floor, e.g. to go to lunch, etc.

II. Intra-Operative Period

   A. "Holding Area" - Dimly lit special area near Operating Room and remain here until surgeon is ready.
     . O.R. staff in attendance, <u>not left alone</u>.

   B. Recovery Room (PAR) - Brightly lit area that all patients having a general anesthetic go to after surgery until awake and reacting.
     . Vital signs checked frequently.

III. Post-Operative Period-Indicate in blank provided explanation given to patient.

   A. Post-op regime.

     1. Diet _____

     2. Activity_____

     3. Special Treatments or Checks_____

     4. Restrictions, if any_____

     5. Exercises: Breathing_____Extremities_____

     6. Specialized Instructions for Patient_____

     7. Pain Medication_____

IV. Fears, misconceptions, or need for more information expressed?

   _____

   _____

V. General response to teaching; cooperation with demonstration.

   _____

   _____

For more information, phone 9-263-3100 and request tape number G1038 (Before and After Surgery).

Figure 3-1. Preoperative teaching guide. (Courtesy Madison General Hospital, Madison, WI)

pleural pressure, and the greater the pressure gradient from positive to negative, the greater the volume of inhaled air.

Increasing transpulmonary pressure helps maintain alveolar expansion. But to prevent recollapse, the alveoli must not only be hyperinflated, but also held open for at least 3 seconds (alveolar inflation time). Techniques achieving these two objectives include: incentive spirometry, voluntary deep breathing, sighing, and yawning.

Incentive Spirometry

An incentive spirometer helps the patient take slow deep breaths. By generating high transpulmonary pressures it produces increased lung volume with an adequate alveolar inflation time. Additionally, the increased transpulmonary pressure enhances venous return.

Incentive spirometers measure the patient's efforts in either flow or volume. Both maintain muscle strength and promote pulmonary hygiene. A flow incentive spirometer, such as illustrated in Figure 3-2, measures the flow rate in cubic centimeters per second, and the patient receives immediate feedback about the amount of air inspired. When the patient generates an adequate flow rate one or more balls or other objects float upward. To calculate the amount of air inhaled, multiply the ml/sec of flow by the duration in seconds of inspiration.

Some flow incentive spirometers allow changes to be made in the flow requirements. That is, the amount of effort the patient must expend can be changed. Since incentive spirometers do not have a device that "locks in" the volume, the nurse instructs the patient not to change the preset volume.

Volume incentive spirometers measure pulmonary exercise more precisely than flow incentive spirometers and calculate volume from flow. Since volume incentive spirometers are more complex than flow incentive spirometers, they are appropriate for the patient who has two or more pulmonary risk factors and is undergoing major surgery.

Despite the plethora of incentive spirometers, most are only as beneficial as the person supervising their use. Therefore, the nurse not only supervises the patient's use postoperatively, but also instructs him in its proper use preoperatively. A return demonstration helps the nurse evaluate the effectiveness of her teaching and also provides baseline data that will allow her to compare the patient's pre- and postoperative efforts.

When instructing the preoperative patient to use an incentive spirometer, the nurse tells him to

> Hold the spirometer upright.
> Keep the ball raised for the count of three.
> Use the spirometer at least 10 times during each waking hour.
> Avoid using the spirometer around mealtime.

The patient should hold the spirometer upright, because tilting it toward himself decreases the effort required to raise the ball. Although tilting the spirometer makes it easier to use, the resulting decrease in effort does not build respiratory strength. The patient must keep the ball raised for the count of three to achieve a given volume. To maintain alveolar inflation, the patient must use the spirometer every hour while he is awake.

The first 5 postoperative days, the patient performs incentive spirometery at least 10 times during each waking hour. To avoid becoming overtired, he takes 5 normal breaths between each attempt. The flow or volume is increased progressively, and the patient's technique, frequency of use, and goal attainment reassessed. The nurse instructs the patient not to use the

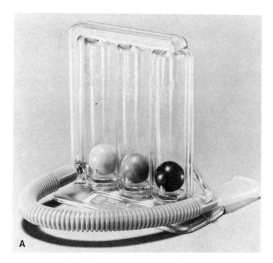

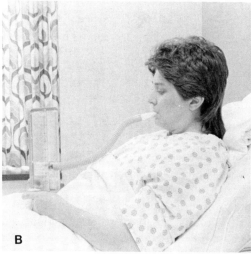

Figure 3-2. Flow-incentive spirometer (A). (Courtesy Chesebrough-Pond.) Positioning of client during administration of incentive spirometry (B). Head of bed should be elevated to at least a 45-degree angle.

incentive spirometer immediately before or after meals, because it may cause nausea.

Voluntary Deep Breathing, Sighing, and Yawning

Deep breathing, sighing, and yawning all hyperventilate the alveoli and prevent their recollapse. Deep breathing, sighing, and yawning also facilitate the even distribution of surfactant in the lungs.

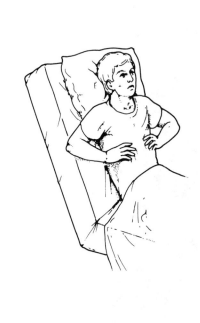

Procedure for Deep Breathing

1. Lie in a semi-Fowler's position, with the neck and back supported

2. Rest hands lightly on front of rib cage. Feeling his chest rise will tell the patient that his lungs are expanding

3. Exhale gently and completely

4. Inhale through the nose as deeply and gently as possible (Gentle inspiration allows blocked or collapsed alveoli to accept air.)

5. Hold this breath and count to three

6. Exhale as completely as possible

7. Repeat 3 times

8. Do this exercise every hour the first postoperative day
Frequency thereafter depends on the patient's risk factors and progress

To deep breathe the patient takes a deep breath to *total lung capacity* and holds it for 3 seconds. The proper procedure for deep breathing is illustrated above.

Normally a person sighs every 5 to 10 minutes, taking in between 1000 cc and 1500 cc of air. However, postoperative patients do not sigh, so the nurse encourages them to do so.

Yawning, a spontaneous deep inspiration, can be initiated by suggestion. The nurse can ask the patient to yawn, discuss yawning, or yawn herself. Ideally, the patient inhales twice before exhaling the first breath.

Coughing

While voluntary sustained maximal inspiration is consistently effective in inflating alveoli, expiratory maneuvers such as forced coughing and the use of blow bottles are not. They can cause the pleural pressure to exceed the airway pressure, and the alveoli deflate and collapse. Furthermore, expiratory maneuvers, unlike inspiratory exercises, are painful. However, since coughing will be necessary if the patient's lungs become congested, the nurse teaches him to cough effectively before surgery. Surgical procedures contraindicating postoperative coughing include ear and eye surgery, neurosurgery, and repair of hiatal and large abdominal hernias.

If the patient will have an abdominal or upper thoracic incision, he needs to know how to cough without creating excessive tension on the incision. The nurse teaches him one of several techniques. The patient can stick out his tongue when he coughs. Or, he can sit in a semi-Fowler's position with his knees bent and support the incision with a pillow, a folded bath blanket, or interlaced fingers, as illustrated below.

The patient may be afraid to cough, deep breathe, or move because he believes that his incision will "come apart." The nurse reassures him that the sutures are very secure and coordinates his attempts at coughing with the administration of pain medication. This means that the nurse must be aware of the onset, peak action, and duration of postoperative pain medications. In addition, she must be aware of a patient's response to pain and pain medications.

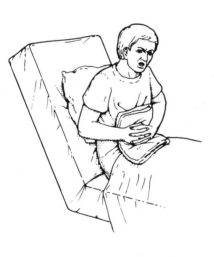

Procedure to Splint an Abdominal Incision and To Cough

1. Lean forward from a semi-Fowler's position, or sit with feet supported to decrease tension on abdominal muscles

2. Place a pillow, folded bath blanket, or interlaced fingers across an abdominal incision to splint it

3. Inhale deeply and slowly through the nose and exhale through the mouth, three times

4. Take a deep breath and hold it for 3 seconds

5. "Hack out" sharply for 3 short breaths

6. With mouth open, quickly take a deep breath

7. Immediately cough deeply once or twice

8. Repeat this exercise once or twice

9. Follow coughing with another maximal deep breath to reinflate collapsed lung areas

Body Movement

Other interventions also help prevent postoperative pulmonary complications. Unless contraindicated by the surgery, these interventions include: assisting the patient to a modified sitting position, which improves ventilation and perfusion matching in the lung; helping him turn from side to side at least every 2 hours, which helps loosen lung secretions; performing passive leg exercises; encouraging him to exercise his legs, and helping him to walk as soon as possible. Illustrated on the following pages are the proper procedures for turning from side to side, getting out of bed, and actively exercising leg muscles, respectively. The nurse assures the patient preoperatively that she will make it as painless as possible for him to turn from side to side, move, and get out of bed by giving pain medication in advance.

To be effective, postoperative exercises must be done properly and regularly. Therefore, preoperatively the nurse demonstrates an exercise and asks the patient for a return demonstration. Postoperatively, exercises must be done at least every 2 hours to be effective. Therefore, the nurse reinforces preoperative instructions and frequently encourages the patient.

Pain Relief Techniques

The vast majority of patients experience pain after surgery. Postoperative pain can be frightening and can adversely affect a patient's recovery. It not only causes discomfort and anxiety, but also contributes to the development of pulmonary complications.

Preoperatively the nurse explains the interventions that will be used to relieve the pain. She also describes the sensations that the patient may experience and the measures that will be used to minimize distressing and painful situations. The nurse instructs the patient to ask for pain medication when he needs it and not to wait until the pain becomes severe. The nurse advises the patient to intercept the pain and not to endure it. The patient suffers less, is less anxious, and is more in control of his discomfort.[6,7] As an important reminder, research has found that nurses tend to undermedicate postoperative patients.[7]

If an electronic pain control device or epidural narcotics will be used, the nurse explains them. Additionally, she demonstrates and asks for a return demonstration of noninvasive techniques such as distraction and relaxation.

Preoperatively the nurse assesses the patient's pain experience. She explores his experience with pain and ascertains the amount of discomfort he expects postoperatively. She asks him to describe the pain he experienced with previous surgeries and the pain relief techniques that were effective. If the patient has not had previous surgery, the nurse asks him how he copes with a headache or backache.

The nurse also assesses the type of anxiety to which the patient is prone. Trait anxiety is a personality characteristic that increases the fear of generally threatening experiences. Based in the patient's social, cultural and religious background, trait anxiety stems from complex psychological factors.

Procedures for Turning

To Turn From Side to Side

1. Raise one knee, planting foot firmly on the mattress; place the arm opposite the raised leg overhead in the direction of the turn and grasp the side rail

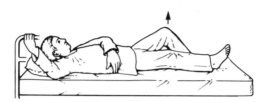

2. Roll onto side, pushing with the bent leg and pulling on the side rail

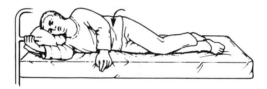

To Turn Back

1. Bend the knee of the upper leg; place palm of hand firmly on the mattress

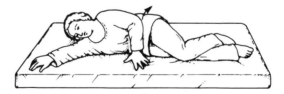

2. Push over onto back

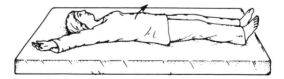

Procedure for Getting Out of Bed

Repeat the steps for turning side to side (without use of a guardrail).

1. Place palms of hands on bed

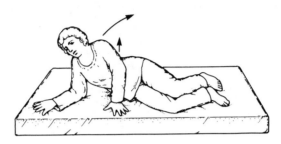

2. Push self up sideways while swinging feet and legs out of bed

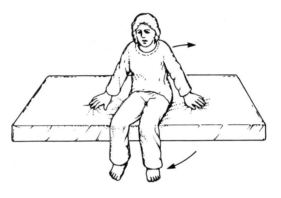

State anxiety is a transient emotional response to a specific threatening experience. While normally not afraid, the patient is now fearful because of a current event such as impending surgery.

The patient with high levels of trait anxiety may need more pain medication postoperatively. While postoperative pain is not greater, its emotional impact is.

Preoperative Medical Orders

Nutrition

Several factors affect a patient's dietary orders preoperatively. Three such factors are the type of anesthesia to be used, the surgical procedure to be done, and the patient's nutritional status.

Procedure To Exercise Leg Muscles

1. Lie in a semi-Fowler's position and bend the knee, raise the foot, and keep it elevated for a few seconds

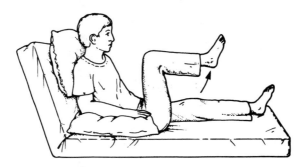

2. Extend the lower leg

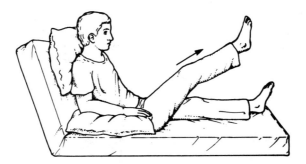

3. Lower the leg to the bed. Do this 5 times with one leg, then repeat with the other leg

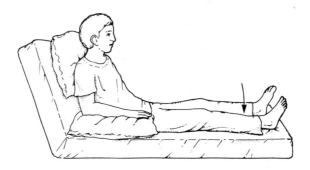

(Continued)

4. Point the toes of both feet toward the foot of the bed. Relax both feet

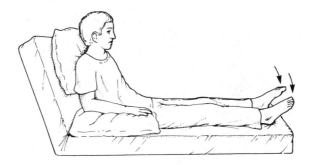

5. Pull toes toward the chin. Relax both feet

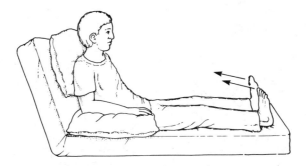

6. Make circles with both ankles. First circle to the right, then to the left. Repeat 3 times. Relax feet

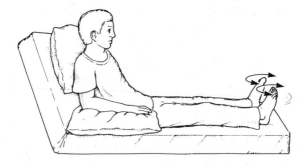

If general anesthesia is to be given, a patient's diet does not usually change until the day before surgery. For elective surgery, solid foods are omitted 12 hours preoperatively and fluids 8 hours preoperatively. This helps avoid aspiration of gastric contents if the patient vomits while anesthetized.

Aspiration is a serious problem. It can lead to pneumonia and has a mortality rate of 50% to 90%, depending upon the amount of gastric contents aspirated. Therefore, if the patient has not been NPO for 4 to 8 hours preoperatively, the surgeon and/or anesthesiologist should be notified. Surgery may need to be rescheduled.

The same NPO criteria apply for major regional anesthesia. For if the block is inadequate, a general anesthetic must be quickly substituted and the stomach should be empty. However, if a patient is to have a local or spinal anesthetic, he may be allowed to eat a light meal 2 to 3 hours before surgery.

Special Orders

Special orders are written for the patient scheduled for bowel surgery, for the diabetic patient, and for the malnourished patient. A patient undergoing bowel surgery may be placed on a low-residue diet preoperatively.

Diabetics scheduled for surgery are usually admitted at least 1 to 2 days in advance. Several routines are used to manage type I diabetics. Each routine, however, begins on the day of surgery. The patient's usual breakfast may be replaced with an infusion of 5% dextrose in water, saline, or Ringer's lactate. In the two most accepted routines, the patient's usual intermediate and/or long-acting insulin is eliminated and regular insulin is administered according to blood glucose results.

For type II diabetics who are going to have major surgery and who will be receiving a general anesthesia, the oral hypoglycemic agent is discontinued well in advance. Since chlorpropamide (Diabinese) has a 36-hour half-life, it must be discontinued a full 3 days preoperatively. If the surgery is less serious, the oral hypoglycemic is discontinued once the patient is NPO and is resumed once he begins to eat. On the day of surgery, intravenous feedings are started with 5% dextrose in water, saline, or Ringer's lactate.

If a patient is malnourished and able to eat preoperatively, a high-protein, high-carbohydrate diet is ordered. This helps ensure adequate nutrition that minimizes those postoperative complications associated with poor nutrition, such as wound infection. The nurse makes sure that the patient can eat those foods on his dietary tray. She also makes sure that patients needing dentures to eat have them in place, and she assists patients needing help.

Total Parenteral Nutrition

Total parenteral nutrition (TPN) is used preoperatively with several groups of patients. These include those who cannot eat, should not eat, will not eat, cannot eat enough, or who have special metabolic problems. Total parenteral nutrition is used successfully, for example, with malnourished patients requiring prolonged periods of bowel preparation prior to diagnostic studies and major surgical procedures. It provides adequate nutrition for as long as necessary when use of the gastrointestinal tract is contraindicated. It keeps the bowel free of particulate matter and greatly reduces colonic bacteria, even when antibiotics are not administered.

Malnourished surgical patients are in high-risk morbidity and mortality categories if surgery is performed before their nutritional status is improved. Therefore, TPN is used to reduce the urgency for surgery in patients in whom prolonged malnutrition has significantly increased the risk of surgery.

TPN also helps avoid, reduce, or correct protein deficiencies and the complications associated with hypoproteinemia. The infusion of amino acids and caloric substrates provides proteins that are required both for repair and restoration of injured tissues. Protein supplementation achieves numerous goals, as listed:

1. Increases resistance to blood loss
2. Decreases the susceptibility to shock
3. Restores serum and tissue proteins
4. Increases plasma and blood volume
5. Increases resistance to infection
6. Reduces edema both locally at the wound and generally
7. Accelerates wound healing
8. Restores digestive enzymes to normal
9. Reverses the protein deficiency of malabsorption
10. Improves metabolic rate
11. Improves cardiovascular function
12. Decreases weakness and lassitude
13. Reverses mental depression
14. Reduces morbidity and mortality
15. Reduces time and expense of convalescence[8]

The basic nutrient mixture of intravenous hyperalimentation solution is listed in Table 3-2. One liter of this solution provides approximately 1000 calories and about 6.5 gm to 8.0 gm of nitrogen, which is equivalent to 40 gm to 50 gm of protein.

Fluids and Electrolytes

Fluid and electrolyte deficiencies must be corrected preoperatively, and patients may be hydrated with crystalloid or colloid intravenous fluids. For example, patients undergoing a major vascular procedure in which adequate renal perfusion is essential and patients who are relatively hypovolemic will be hydrated with crystalloid solution.

Blood may be administered preoperatively to alleviate serious blood volume depletion resulting either from acute or from chronic diseases or to reach optimum hemoglobin and hematocrit levels advocated for surgical patients. Research suggests that a hemoglobin level of 10 g/dl ensures maximum tissue oxygen supply. At this level ventricular force and ventricular blood supply are normal. In addition, the decrease in blood viscosity may be beneficial.

Table 3-2
Adult Intravenous Hyperalimentation Solution

Base Solution	
40–50% dextrose in water	500 ml
8.5–10% crystalline amino acids	500 ml
Additives to Each Unit	
Sodium chloride	40–50 mEq
Potassium chloride	20–30 mEq
Potassium acid phosphate (10–20 mM phosphorus)	15–30 mEq
Magnesium sulfate	15–18 mEq
Additives to Any One Unit Daily	
Calcium gluconate 10%	4.5 mEq
Multivitamin infusion (MVI–12)	10 ml
Zinc sulfate	5 mg
Copper sulfate	1–2 mg
Iron-dextran (Imferon)	0.1 ml
Chromium chloride	1.5 mcg
Manganese chloride	0.5 mg
Selenium (Na_2SeO_3)	60.0 mcg
Additive to Any One Unit Twice Weekly	
Vitamin K	10 mg
Intravenous Fat Emulsion 10% or 20%	
500 ml 2–7 times weekly over 4–6 hr	50–100 gm
Carbohydrate calories	850 kcal/liter
Protein calories	150 kcal/liter
Fat calories	500–1000 kcal/liter
Nitrogen	6.5–8.0 gm/liter
Amino acids	40–50 gm/liter

Dudrick SJ: Parenteral nutrition. In Dudrick SJ, et al. (eds): Manual of Preoperative and Postoperative Care, 3rd ed, p 95. Philadelphia, WB Saunders, 1983

A hematocrit of 33% is thought to be optimal for the critically ill, general surgical patient. Blood may be administered to increase oxygen availability if the hematocrit is below 33%. However, hemoglobin and hematocrit are not always normalized before surgery. For example, patients whose surgery requires the use of cardiopulmonary bypass do better immediately postoperatively with some degree of hemodilution.

If blood is administered, surgery is ideally postponed a day to allow the blood volume to readjust. In addition, the transfused red blood cells need time to accumulate a normal level of 2,3-diphosphoglycerate (2,3-DPG), which is necessary for the efficient delivery of oxygen to the tissues.

Gastrointestinal Intubation

A variety of situations necessitate insertion of a nasogastric tube. The situation dictates when it will be inserted.

The tube will be inserted preoperatively if the patient has a gastrointestinal obstruction or ileus with possible gastric residual. Gastric intubation decreases the possibility of vomiting and aspiration during induction of anesthesia.

A nasogastric tube will be inserted intraoperatively if peristalsis will decrease or stop postoperatively because of manipulation of the intestines during surgery. A nasogastric tube will also be inserted during surgery to protect a suture line if gastric or esophageal surgery has been performed.

Bowel Preparation

Bowel preparations are not routinely done preoperatively and when they are, the extent of the preparation depends upon the type and site of surgery. For example, if the patient is going to be confined to bed several days postoperatively and has not had a bowel movement within the past day or two, a mild laxative or Fleet enema may be ordered. This empties the lower gastrointestinal tract, preventing postoperative constipation and fecal impaction. Similarly, enemas and cathartics are given following preoperative barium studies to avoid postoperative obstruction and fecal impaction.

A more extensive bowel preparation is ordered for the patient undergoing surgery on the gastrointestinal tract, pelvis, perineum, or rectum. Preoperative enemas help empty the bowel, thus minimizing injury to the colon, and providing better visualization of the operative site.

Preoperative bowel preparation for patients undergoing elective colon surgery is imperative. Since the colon lumen must be entered during surgery, escaping bacteria can invade adjacent tissues and cause serious infections. Therefore, preoperative preparation includes a mechanical bowel prep and the oral administration of antimicrobials. Cathartics and enemas remove gross collections of stool, and oral antimicrobial therapy suppresses potent microflora without inducing overgrowth of resistant strains.

Since it is desirable to suppress both aerobic and anaerobic intestinal microorganisms, a combination of antimicrobials is administered the day before surgery. Although the drugs used depend on the surgeon's preference, a typical combination is neomycin and erythromycin. When these drugs are given in 3 doses, for example, at 1 PM, 2 PM, and 11 PM, a minimal level of antibiotic remains in the lumen of the small bowel by the time surgery begins. Therefore, prophylactic antibiotics must be administered at the scheduled times.

Antibiotic enemas may be ordered preoperatively to decrease intestinal bacteria. Since the decrease in bacteria may inhibit the synthesis of vitamin K and predispose the patient to postoperative bleeding, supplementary vitamin K may be given.

Both oral and rectal antibiotics are an adjunct to an adequate mechanical bowel preparation. Since any stool left in the colon because of inadequate and improper cleansing can lead to sepsis, the nurse must make sure that enemas promote complete evacuation of stool.

Enemas " 'til clear" are usually ordered and the physician should be notified if the results are not clear after the third enema. Some physicians order up to three enemas the evening before surgery and if the results are not clear, will order additional enemas to be given the next morning. The nurse must be aware that fluid and electrolyte imbalances, such as fluid excess and potassium depletion, can result when enemas are given until the results are clear. Patients at risk for fluid and electrolyte imbalances are the elderly and those who have been NPO for tests but have not been receiving intravenous fluids.

Vaginal Preparation

A medicated douche may be ordered preoperatively to cleanse the perineal area if a patient is going to have gynecologic or urologic surgery. For example, a douche may be ordered for a patient scheduled for a hysterectomy.

Urinary Preparation

Urinary retention can occur postoperatively due to overdistention and loss of bladder tone. Overdistention causes bladder atonicity and anticholinergics, such as atropine, can cause loss of bladder tone. To avoid postoperative urinary retention, a patient undergoing a short procedure is usually asked to urinate before being medicated. However, certain urologic procedures, such as a cystoscopy, require urine in the bladder.

In certain situations an indwelling catheter is inserted either just before the patient is transported to the operating room or after he is anesthetized. An indwelling catheter is needed when the patient is undergoing a prolonged procedure, when bladder distention will interfere with exposure in the pelvis, for example, during abdominoperineal resection, and when the patient's urinary output must be monitored hourly.

Skin Preparation

The skin is the body's first line of defense against invading microorganisms, and any break in the skin is a potential portal of infection. Therefore, the skin is carefully prepared preoperatively so as to rid the operative site of as many microorganisms as possible.

When surgery is elective, the patient washes the operative site with a soap containing a detergent-germicide for several days preoperatively. And ideally, the day of surgery, the patient takes a warm bath or shower using Betadine soap. If an early morning surgery is scheduled, the patient bathes or showers the night before, which reduces the number of skin organisms.

The Immediate Preoperative Period

Patient Reassessment and Preparation

The patient should be allowed to sleep as long as possible the morning of surgery. Sleeplessness, fatigue, and anxiety are to be avoided in the preoperative patient because they have been reported to enhance the stress response, *i.e.,* adrenocortical activity. The patient may have been given a sedative the night before the day of surgery to ensure a good night's rest. Any additional sedatives or pain medications must have been given at least 4 hours before the preoperative medication.

Approximately 60 to 90 minutes before surgery is scheduled, the nurse reassesses the patient. Completion of a preoperative checklist, such as illustrated in Figure 3-3, ensures that the nurse does not overlook any aspect of care and facilitates documentation of her interventions.

Vital signs are documented on the checklist. They will provide valuable information for both the operating and postanesthesia recovery room staff. Additionally, the patient's height and weight will be helpful.

The nurse checks the patient's identaband to make sure that the patient's name is clear and legible. The band must be securely attached, since the operating room staff use it to identify the patient.

The nurse also notes on the checklist where the patient's family will be waiting. Similarly, the family must know where the surgeon plans to meet them. Families frequently wait long hours to learn the outcome of a surgery, and it is extremely frustrating for them to "just miss" the doctor. Some surgeons meet the patient's family in the surgical waiting room after the surgery to discuss the procedure and the patient's condition. Frequently volunteers staff the room. They provide quiet reassurance and answer the telephone when the recovery room nurse calls to announce the patient's arrival. Other surgeons prefer to meet the patient's family in the patient's room.

The nurse notes any handicaps that the patient has and any special precautions to be taken. Patient conditions such as an immobile joint and lack of subcutaneous fat affect how the patient is moved and positioned on the operating table.

The patient is asked to void unless he has a urologic condition or an indwelling catheter. The time that he voids is documented on the checklist.

Articles that could be lost or damaged in the operating room, such as jewelry, wigs, and prostheses, are removed. However, a plain wedding band can be taped to the patient's finger. Similarly, when a patient prefers not to be seen without a wig, it is removed after the patient is anesthetized and is returned to the patient's room. One prosthesis that is NOT removed is a hearing aid. In fact, the nurse makes absolutely certain that the surgical and recovery room staff know that the patient has a hearing aid in place.

Hairpins are removed because they might injure the patient's head. Long hair is braided so that it will not become tangled or interfere with equipment.

Date:

Surgical Procedure Scheduled:

Allergies:

O.R. NURSE CHECK | UNIT NURSE CHECK

14. _____   14. Voided: _____
      Yes or No   Time

1. _____   1. Identaband checked: _____
      Yes or No

15. _____   15. Retention Catheter: _____
      Yes or No

2. _____   2. Consent for surgery signed: _____
      Yes or No

16. _____   16.   None   Removed
      Wigs _____
      Hair Pins _____
      Nail Polish _____
      Make-Up _____
      Jewelry _____

3. _____   3. History & Physical: _____
      Yes or No

4. _____   4. Note by Surgeon: Yes or No

17. _____   17. Dentures: None   Removed
      Bridge _____
      Partial _____
      Plates _____

5. _____   5. NPO Since _____
      Time

6. _____   6. Condition when leaving for surgery: (circle)

      Oriented, Drowsy, Asleep, Non-responsive, Very Restless, Apprehensive, Disoriented, Very Talkative.

Eyes:
      Artificial _____
      Contacts _____

Other Prothesis: _____

7. _____   7. Type & Crossmatch:
      No. units available _____
      Not ordered _____
      Being done _____

18. _____   18. Pre-op Blood Pressure: _____

19. _____   19. Pre-op Hypo: _____
      Type   Time

8. _____   8. Anti-embolism stockings:
      On _____
      Not ordered _____

Other Medication(s): _____
      Type   Time

9. _____   9. Family: Absent _____
      4C Surgical Waiting _____
      At This Number _____
      Other _____

      Type   Time

Signature: O.R. R.N.   Signature: Unit R.N.

10. _____   10. Handicaps or Special Precautions: (Circle)

      Immobile Joint, Paralysis, Diabetic, Infections, Speech & Hearing Disorders (describe), Blind, None.

11. _____   11. Urinalysis   Results on Chart _____
      CBC   Spec. to Lab _____
      Not Done _____

PERMANENT - MAINTAIN WITH RECORD

12. _____   12. Chest X-ray   Results on Chart _____
      Done _____
      Not Ordered _____

13. _____   13. ECG   Results on Chart _____
      Done _____
      Not Ordered _____

Figure 3-3. Preoperative checklist. (Courtesy Madison General Hospital, Madison, WI)

The patient is also asked to remove nail polish and makeup. They make it difficult to assess the color of the patient's nailbeds and skin. Both are observed to assess adequacy of circulation and the development of hypoxemia.

Dentures are removed preoperatively because they can cause respiratory obstruction during anesthesia. If loose, the dentures can fall away from the gums and drop into the pharynx when the jaw muscles relax. If a patient does not wish to be seen without dentures, they can be removed in the surgical reception area and returned to the patient's room.

Preoperative Medication

Preoperative or preanesthesia medications are administered for a variety of reasons. They allay anxiety, permit a smoother induction of anesthesia, decrease the amount of anesthesia needed, create amnesia for the events that precede surgery, and minimize the flow of pharyngeal and respiratory secretions. In addition, some sedatives used for preoperative medication reduce the stress response caused by preoperative emotional stressors. Pentobarbital, hydroxyzine, and diazepam all inhibit adrenocortical stimulation. Meperidine, however, does not. The nurse explains that, depending upon what has been ordered, the medications may cause a dry mouth, and that, while not used to induce sleep, they aid in relaxation, and may cause drowsiness.

The types of agents that may be administered include anticholinergics (vagolytics or drying agents), sedatives, tranquilizers, antianxiety agents, narcotic analgesics, neuroleptanalgesic agents, and cimetidine. The type and amount of premedication ordered depends upon a number of factors, one of which is the patient's age. For example, while infants usually receive only atropine, adults receive a combination of agents, depending upon body size. Dosages are reduced for the debilitated or elderly patient, and some anesthesiologists prefer to prescribe only tranquilizers for elderly patients. The potential hypotension that may result from these drugs is less dangerous than the severe respiratory depression that may accompany opiates. Table 3-3 identifies the most commonly used preoperative medications.

Anticholinergics (vagolytic or drying agents) include medications such as atropine, glycopyrrolate (Robinul), and scopolamine. By decreasing pulmonary and oropharyngeal secretions, these agents minimize operative and postoperative secretions. However, in addition to minimizing operative and postoperative secretions, these agents also obtund vagal reflexes that could cause fatal cardiac dysrhythmias if induced during anesthesia and surgery. In some centers vagolytic or drying agents are used less frequently today because newer anesthetics make secretions less of a problem. (Note: Anticholinergics are a holdover from the "ether days" but still are used as a routine in most places.)

Sedatives, tranquilizers, and antianxiety agents such as sodium pentobarbital, secobarbital, diazepam, and hydroxyzine hydrochloride generally make induction of anesthesia smoother and more efficient. They alleviate the patient's anxiety and apprehension.

Narcotic analgesics such as morphine and meperidine hydrochloride sedate the patient and help him relax before induction. They are not given to reduce postoperative pain, but rather to minimize the patient's perception of pain. In addition, these agents decrease the amount of anesthetic needed. Therefore, if these medications are not given at the time ordered by the anesthesiologist or surgeon, the person who ordered them should be notified.

Neuroleptanalgesic agents such as Innovar are newer preparations that are gaining popularity. They result in a general state of calmness and somnolence without total unconsciousness.

Table 3-3
Commonly Used Preoperative Medications

Medication	Usual Adult Dose	Desired Effects	Undesired Effects
Anticholinergics			
atropine	0.4–0.6 mg	Decreases oral, respiratory, and gastric secretions, thus facilitating intubation. Prevents laryngospasms. Prevents reflex bradycardia	Excessive dryness of the mouth; Tachycardia; flushing Increased ocular tension, blurred vision, dilated pupils Restlessness, excitability, and confusion possibly progressing to anticholinergic intoxication May cause urinary retention
glycopyrrolate (Robinul)	0.002 mg/pound	Same as for atropine, but decreases oral secretions more effectively	Same as for atropine, but does not cross the blood brain barrier so CNS effects are usually absent
scopolamine hydrobromide	0.4–0.6 mg	Same as for atropine	Same as for atropine
Sedatives-Hypnotics			
pentobarbital sodium (Nembutal Sodium)	50–200 mg	Reduces anxiety Promotes relaxation and sleep	May cause confusion or excitement in the elderly or in patients with severe pain No analgesic effect
secobarbital sodium (Seconal Sodium)	50–200 mg	Same as for pentobarbital	Same as for pentobarbital
Tranquilizers			
promethazine	25–50 mg	Reduces anxiety	Postoperative hypotension

(continued)

Table 3-3 (Continued)
Commonly Used Preoperative Medications

Medication	Usual Adult Dose	Desired Effects	Undesired Effects
Tranquilizers (continued) hydrochloride (Phenergan)		Antiemetic	
chlorpromazine (Thorazine)	12.5–25 mg	Same as for promethazine	Same as for promethazine
Antianxiety Agents diazepam (Valium)	5–10 mg	Provides sedation and amnesia Reduces anxiety and apprehension	Respiratory depression Excessive sedation Preoperative or postoperative nausea and vomiting
hydroxyzine hydrochloride (Vistaril)	25–100 mg	Reduces anxiety Antiemetic	Drowsiness and dry mouth
Narcotics meperidine hydrochloride (Demerol)	50–100 mg	Reduces anxiety, promotes relaxation Minimizes perception of pain Decreases amount of anesthetic needed Produces sedation	Depresses respiration, circulation, and gastric motility Dizziness, tachycardia, and sweating Hypotension, restlessness, and excitement Preoperative or postoperative nausea and vomiting
morphine sulfate	5–10 mg	Same as for meperidine	Same as for meperidine

Neuroleptanalgesic Agent			
fentanyl and droperidol (Innovar)	0.5–2.0 ml	General calmness, state of indifference	Respiratory depression; hypotension; muscle rigidity
		Decreases motor activity	Occasional restlessness and dysphoria (will refuse to go to surgery)
		Analgesia	Outer tranquility with inner turmoil
		Antiemetic	
Antihistamines (H_2 Receptor)			
cimetidine (Tagamet)	300 mg	Decreases gastric acidity and volume	Decreased clearance of other drugs including diazepam, lidocaine, and propranolol
ranitidine (Zantac)	150 mg	Same as cimetidine	Same as cimetidine

Cimetidine and the newer drug, ranitidine, are H_2 blockers being increasingly advocated for use preoperatively. They decrease both gastric acidity and volume. Therefore, if the patient vomits and aspirates, a much milder pneumonitis results than if he aspirates gastric contents with a pH of less than 2.5. These medications are usually given the evening before surgery and again some time during the day of surgery.

Patient Safety

Once the nurse has given the preoperative medication, she raises the side rails. In addition, if the patient has a hiatal hernia or reflux, she elevates the head of the bed. She instructs the patient to stay in bed and to press the call light for help.

A family member or significant other may wish to visit the patient before surgery, perhaps even accompanying him to the doors of the operating room. Although the patient is to be quiet and calm preoperatively, he may find the presence of a loved one comforting.

The patient is usually transported to the surgical reception area on a stretcher but sometimes may be moved in bed. The person transporting the patient tells the nurse that he is ready to take the patient to the operating room, and the nurse helps the transporter move the patient from his bed to the stretcher. The nurse checks the patient's identification band and chart one more time to make sure that everything has been done and documented. Then, before the patient leaves the room, the nurse makes certain that the side rails are raised, the seat belts are securely fastened, the patient is adequately covered, and that he knows when he will see his family.

The Surgical Reception Area

In some hospitals, the surgical reception or holding area is a separate room near the surgical suite. It is quiet and may have facilities for preparing the incisional site, starting intravenous infusions, inserting catheters, and administering medications. Patients are placed head first in the surgical reception area. Being able to see approaching staff affords patients some control over their environment.

The registered nurse who staffs the surgical reception area greets and cares for patients while the operating suite is being prepared. The knowledge and skills of the nurse enable her to assess the patient and his needs and to intervene appropriately. The nurse verifies the information documented on the Preoperative Checklist and notifies the appropriate person should she find discrepancies or omissions.

The nurse assesses the patient, integrating her data with that gleaned from the preoperative assessment and documented on the Nursing History and Preoperative Teaching Guide. The nurse reassures the patient, helps calm his fears and anxieties, and documents her findings and actions.

When the circulating nurse arrives to transport the patient to the operating suite, the nurse in the surgical reception area conveys significant patient information to her. A compilation of data representing preoperative assessment, preoperative preparation, and the assessment conducted during the patient's stay in the surgical reception area, this information provides a comprehensive view of the patient's perioperative experience to date.

After introducing herself to the patient, the circulating nurse transfers him to the operating suite. The supplies have been opened, and the surgeon is scrubbing, because once in the suite, the patient is and must be the center of attention.

Evaluation

The patient is physically and emotionally prepared for the surgical procedure and events of the intra- and postoperative periods.

Summary

Preoperative preparation begins when the patient is admitted to the hospital. The nurse uses data gleaned from the preoperative assessment and from subsequent reassessments to tailor preoperative preparation. Although surgical procedure and medical care dictate some aspects of preoperative preparation, the patient himself and factors that make him unique suggest others. Therefore, the nurse skillfully and knowledgeably incorporates prescribed medical orders into a patient care plan that meets the needs of the patient. Outcome criteria appropriate for a patient in the preoperative phase are listed below.

Outcome Criteria for a Patient in the Preoperative Phase

1. The patient coughs effectively and maintains a clear airway
2. The patient remains oriented to person, place, and time
3. The patient's nutritional intake is adequate to meet his needs
4. Physical and emotional factors increasing the patient's risk for surgery have been evaluated
5. The patient is physically and emotionally prepared for surgery
6. The patient correctly demonstrates how to turn, cough, deep breathe, splint his incision, and get out of bed
7. The patient explains how his pain will be controlled postoperatively
8. The patient correctly explains anticipated events of the intra- and postoperative phases
9. The patient has signed the operative permit

References

1. Johnson JE: Stress reduction through sensation information. In Sarason IG, Spielberger CH (eds): Stress and Anxiety, Vol. 2. New York, Halsted Press, 1976
2. Johnson JE et al: Altering patients' responses to surgery: An extension and replication. Nurs Res, Vol 1:111–121, October 1978
3. Johnson JE et al: Sensory information, instruction in a coping strategy, and recovery from surgery. Res Nurs Health, Vol 1:14–17, April 1978
4. King I, Tarsitano B: The effect of structured and unstructured pre-operative teaching: A replication. Nurs Res 31(6):324–329, November/December 1982
5. Petty C: Opinion — A physician's perspective on allaying patients' fears. AORN J; 41(3):537–542, 1985
6. Heidrich G, Perry S: Helping the patient in pain. Am J Nurs 82(12):1828–1833, 1982
7. Cohen FL: Postsurgical pain relief: Patients' status and nurses' medication choices. Pain, Vol 9:265–274, 1980
8. Dudrick SJ: Parenteral nutrition. In Dudrick SJ et al (eds): Manual of Preoperative and Postoperative Care, 3rd ed, pp 90–91. Philadelphia, WB Saunders, 1983

Bibliography

Association of Operating Room Nurses: AORN Standards and Recommended Practices for Perioperative Nursing. Denver, The Association of Operating Room Nurses, 1983

Baesl TJ, Buckley JJ: Preoperative assessment, preparation for operation, and routine postoperative care. Urol Clin North Am 10(1): 3–17, February 1983

Bender JM, Faubion JM: Total parenteral nutrition. AORN J 40(3): 354–365, September 1984

Bland BV, Miracle VA: The no-write way to document preop patient teaching. Nurs 83 13(12): 48–49, 1983

Bovington MM, Spies ME, Troy PJ: Management of the patient with diabetes mellitus during surgery or illness. Nurs Clin North Am 18(4): 661–671, December 1983

Brunner LS, Suddarth DS: Perioperative management of the surgical patient. In Brunner LS, Suddarth DS: Textbook of Medical-Surgical Nursing, 5th ed. Philadelphia, JB Lippincott, 1984

Bullock BL: Physiologic effects of stress. In Bullock BL, Rosendahl PP: Pathophysiology — Adaptations and Alterations in Function. Boston, Little, Brown & Co, 1984

Buzby GP, Mullen JL: Nutrition and the surgical patient. In Goldmann DR et al (eds): Medical Care of the Surgical Patient. Philadelphia, JB Lippincott, 1982

Cahill CA: Yawn maneuver to prevent atelectasis. AORN J 27(5): 1000–1004, April 1978

Carey KW: Caring for Surgical Patients. Springhouse, PA, Intermed Communications, 1982

Carrick L: Considerations for the older surgical patient. Geriatr Nurs 3(1): 43–50, January/February 1982

Cascorbi HF: Perianesthetic problems with nonanesthetic drugs. In Am Soc Anesth Refresher Course, Vol 6, 1978

Cebul RD, Kussmaul WG: Preoperative pulmonary evaluation and preparation. In Goldmann DR et al (eds): Medical Care of the Surgical Patient. Philadelphia, JB Lippincott, 1982

Cerrato PL: Is your patient *really* ready for surgery? RN 48(6): 69–70, 1985

Chansky ER: Reducing patient's anxieties. AORN J 40(3): 375–377, September 1984

Cohen FL: Postsurgical pain relief: Patients' status and nurses' medication choices. Pain, Vol 9: 265–274, 1980

Cohen NH: Three steps to better patient teaching. Nurs 80 10(2): 72–74, 1980

Demling RH: Preoperative care. In Way LW (ed): Current Surgical Diagnosis and Treatment, 6th ed. Los Altos, CA, Lange Medical Publications 1983

Drain CB: Managing postoperative pain — It's a matter of sighs. Nurs 84 14(8):52–55, August 1984

Dudrick SJ: Parenteral nutrition. In Dudrick SJ et al (eds): Manual of Preoperative and Postoperative Care, 3rd ed. Philadelphia, WB Saunders, 1983

Dye L: Surgery. In Guthrie DW, Guthrie RA: Nursing Management of Diabetes Mellitus, 2nd ed. St. Louis, CV Mosby, 1982

Felver L: Understanding the electrolyte maze. Am J Nurs 80(9): 1591–1595, 1980

Folk–Lighty M: Solving the puzzles of patients' fluid imbalances. Nurs 84 14(2): 34–41, 1984

Fraulini KE, Gorski DW: Don't let perioperative medications put you in a spin. Nurs 83 13(12): 26–30, 1983

Fraulini KE, Murphy P: R.E.A.C.T. A new system for measuring postanesthesia recovery. Nurs 84 14(4): 101–102, 1984

Fuchs P: Before and after surgery stay right on respiratory care. Nurs 83 13(5): 47–50, 1983

Garner JS: Guideline for Prevention of Surgical Wound Infections, 1985. Atlanta, U.S. Department of Health and Human Services, Public Health Service and Centers for Disease Control, 1985

Gilmour IJ: Perioperative respiratory care. Urol Clin North Am 10(1): 65–76, February 1983

Glass LB, Jenkins CA: The ups and downs of serum pH. Nurs 83 13(9): 34–41, 1983

Gruendemann BJ, Meeker MH: Alexander's care of the patient. In Surgery, St. Louis, CV Mosby, 1983

Guadagni NP, Hamilton WK: Anesthesiology. In Way LW (ed): Current Surgical Diagnosis and Treatment, 6th ed. Los Altos, CA, Lange Medical Publications, 1983

Heidrich G, Perry S: Helping the patient in pain. Am J Nurs 82(12): 1828–1833, December 1982

Hensle TW: Nutritional support of the surgical patient. Urol Clin North Am 10(1): 109–118, February 1983

Hickey RF: Respiratory disease and the surgical patient. In Way LW (ed): Current Surgical Diagnosis and Treatment, 6th ed. Los Altos, CA, Lange Medical Publications, 1983

Hill GL, Church J: Energy and protein requirements of general surgical patients requiring intravenous nutrition. Br J Surg 71(1): 1–9, 1984

Hudson MF: Drugs and the older adult. Nurs 84 14(8): 47–51, 1984

Huttmann B: Quit wasting time with "nursing rituals". Nurs 85 15(10): 34–39, 1985

Johnson JE: Stress reduction through sensation information. In Sarason IG, Spielberger CH (eds): Stress and Anxiety, Vol. 2. New York, Halsted Press, 1976

Johnson JE et al: Altering patients' responses to surgery: An extension and replication. Nurs Res Vol. 1: 111–121, October 1978

Johnson JE et al: Sensory information, instruction in a coping strategy, and recovery from surgery. Res Nurs Health Vol. 1: 14–17, April 1978

Julien R: Understanding Anesthesia. Menlo Park, CA, Addison–Wesley, 1984

Jung R, Wight J, Nusser R, Rosoff L: Comparison of three methods of respiratory care following upper abdominal surgery. Chest 78(1): 31–35, July 1980

Kee JL: Fluids and Electrolytes with Clinical Applications, 3rd ed. New York, John Wiley & Sons, 1982

Kim MJ, McFarland GK, McLane AM (eds): Pocket Guide to Nursing Diagnoses. St. Louis, CV Mosby, 1984

King I, Tarsitano B: The effect of structured and unstructured pre-operative teaching: A replication. Nurs Res 31(6): 324–329, November/December 1982

Kneedler J, Dodge G: Perioperative Patient Care. Boston, Blackwell Scientific Publications, 1983

Lazarus RS: Emotion and adaptation: Conceptual and empirical relations. In Arnold WJ (ed): Nebraska Symposium on Motivation. Lincoln, University of Nebraska Press, 1968

Lederer DH, Van de Water JM, Indech RB: Which deep breathing device should the postoperative patient use? Chest 77(5): 610–613, 1980

Long BC, Gowin CJ, Bushong ME: Surgical intervention. In Phipps WJ, Long BC, Woods NF(eds): Medical-Surgical Nursing, 2nd ed. St. Louis, CV Mosby, 1983

Mauldin BC: Ambulatory surgery. AORN J 39(5): 770–771, April 1984

McConnell E: Be prepared for double trouble if your surgical patient's a diabetic. Nurs 81 11(11): 118–123, November 1981

McConnell E: How nursing care plans help you. Nurs Life 2(1): 55–59, January/February 1982

McInerney L: Health education. In Howe J, Dickason EJ, Jones DA, Snider MJ (eds): The Handbook of Nursing. New York, John Wiley & Sons, 1984

McNeal P, Duncan ML: Assessing patients in the holding area. Today's OR Nurse 7(3): 16–19, 1985

Meckes PR: Perioperative care of the elderly patient. Today's OR Nurse 6(9): 8–15, 1984

Metheny N: Preoperative fluid balance assessment. AORN J 33(1): 51–56, 1981

Metheny NM: Quick Reference to Fluid Balance. Philadelphia, JB Lippincott, 1984

Metheny MN, Snively Jr WD: Nurses' Handbook of Fluid Balance, 4th ed. Philadelphia, JB Lippincott, 1983

Miller TA, Duke Jr JH: Fluid and electrolyte management. In Dudrick SJ et al (eds): Manual of Preoperative and Postoperative Care, 3rd ed. Philadelphia, WB Saunders, 1983

Nyberg KG: When diabetes complicates your pre- and post-op care. RN 46(1): 42–46, 1983

O'Donohue WJ: National survey of the usage of lung expansion modalities for the prevention and treatment of postoperative atelectasis following abdominal and thoracic surgery. Chest 87(1): 76–80, 1985

O'Donohue WJ: Prevention and treatment of postoperative atelectasis—Can it and will it be adequately studied? Chest 87(1): 1–2, 1985

Ochsner MG: Acute Urinary Retention. Compr Ther 9(8): 61–67, 1983

Pastewski BM, Gerbino PP: Drug reactions and interactions in the surgical patient. In Goldmann DR et al (eds): Medical Care of the Surgical Patient. Philadelphia, JB Lippincott, 1982

Petty C: Opinion—A physician's perspective on allaying patients' fears. AORN J 41(3): 537–542, 1985

Podjasek JH: Which postop patient faces the greatest respiratory risk? RN 48(9): 44–56, 1985

Rankin SH, Duffy, KL: 15 problems in patient education and their solutions. Nurs 84 14(4): 67–81, 1984

Schumann D: Preoperative measures to promote wound healing. Nurs Clin North Am 14(4): 683–699, December 1979

Stock MC, Downs JB, Gauer PK, Alster JM, Imrey PB: Prevention of postoperative pulmonary complications with CPAP, incentive spirometry and conservative therapy. Chest 87(2): 151–157, 1985

Stuhler-Schlag MK: Pre and postoperative fluids and electrolytes. Today's OR Nurse 4(7): 11–15, 66–67, September 1982

Sweeney SS: OR observations: Key to postop pain. AORN J 32(3): 391–400, September 1980

Taylor P: Patient teaching: Keys to more success more often. Nurs Life 2(6): 25–32, November/December 1982

Teasley KM, Lysne J, Nuwer N, Shronts EP, Cerra FB: Nutrition and metabolic support of the surgical patient. Urol Clin North Am 10(1): 119–129, February 1983

Weaver TE: Incentive spirometers. Nurs 81 11(2): 54–58, 1981

Wong J, Wong S: A randomized controlled trail of a new approach to preoperative teaching and patient compliance. Int J Nurs Stud 22(2): 105–115, 1985

Section 2
The Intraoperative Phase

For some must watch while some must sleep.

—Hamlet, Act 3, Scene 2

4 | Patient Positioning

We seek the truth, and will endure the consequences.

—Charles Seymour

Just as the preoperative phase is comprised of numerous events that contribute to a successful outcome for the patient, so is the intraoperative phase comprised of such events. In the intraoperative phase, the patient arrives in the surgical suite where he is positioned on the operating room table, anesthetized, and draped. After the surgical site is properly prepared, the surgery performed, and the wound closed and covered, the patient is transported to the postanesthesia recovery room.

The operating room nurse assesses the patient and reviews the data documented by nurses and other health care professionals who cared for the patient in the preoperative phase. She pays particular attention to factors that increase the patient's risk of surgery. Combining these data with her knowledge of events of the intraoperative phase, she identifies nursing diagnoses such as those listed on page 104. From these diagnoses she derives goals, and develops, implements, and evaluates the plan originally initiated. Additionally, she incorporates any appropriate preoperative interventions that meet the patient's continuing needs.

Nursing Diagnoses Applicable in the Intraoperative Phase

Potential for injury:

    Neuromuscular damage related to improper positioning

    Burns related to improper grounding of electrocautery equipment

    Nosocomial infection

    Related to leaving a foreign object in the wound

Potential for impairment of skin integrity related to improper positioning

Potential for alteration in cardiac output: Decreased cardiac output related to improper positioning

Potential for ineffective breathing pattern related to improper positioning

Potential for alteration in tissue perfusion: Decreased peripheral circulation related to interruption of flow by outside constricting factors.

(From Kim MJ, McFarland GK, McLane AA (eds): Pocket Guide to Nursing Diagnoses. St. Louis, CV Mosby, 1984)

Patient Positioning

Planning for Positioning

Planning for patient positioning intraoperatively begins with the preoperative assessment. Information learned about the patient and existing medical conditions may well affect at what point he is positioned. A patient's limitations, such as an immobile joint, are documented on the Nursing History Form and Preoperative Checklist. The operating room staff uses this information to decide when to position the patient for surgery and to prevent injury to joints and other body parts. For once the patient is anesthetized, his limitations can easily be exceeded and damage done.

Criteria for Positioning

Any position in which a patient is placed for surgery meets certain criteria. The position provides optimum exposure to the operative site and allows the anesthesiologist access for induction of anesthesia and administration of intravenous fluids or drugs. The position promotes circulatory and respiratory function. It promotes the patient's well-being and safety, and therefore avoids excessive pressure on a body part. Additionally, the position facilitates draping in order to ensure the patient's individuality, privacy, and dignity.

Timing of Positioning

When possible, a patient is transferred from the stretcher to the operating room table while awake. Usually the patient is placed in the supine position, anesthetized, and then positioned for surgery. However, if a patient experiences pain upon moving, he may be anesthetized on the stretcher and then moved to the operating room table. Similarly, if a patient is to be placed in the prone position, he may be moved to the operating table and positioned after being anesthetized on the table.

Myriad factors affect when a patient is positioned intraoperatively. Some factors relate specifically to the patient and his physical status, while others pertain to anesthesia and the surgical procedure. Patient parameters include: activity level, age, cardiopulmonary status, central or peripheral nerve dysfunction, metabolic function, muscle tone, pain experienced upon moving, physical disability and its degree, volume status, weight, and the existence of disorders such as arthritis. The anesthetic technique that will be used affects when a patient is positioned, as does the operative site.

Types of Positions

Although a variety of patient positions are used, each is a variation of one of three basic positions: dorsal (supine), prone, or lateral. These basic positions can be modified using special operating room tables and attachments.

No position is risk-free for the sedated and anesthetized patient. However, proper positioning can minimize the resulting physiologic changes and their sequelae. The accompanying display (pages 106 – 113) lists those positions most frequently used in surgery and identifies their use as well as potential problems.

| Evaluation

The patient does not experience any adverse effects as a result of the position in which he was placed during surgery.

| Summary

The position in which the patient is placed intraoperatively depends upon several factors, including the operative procedure and coexisting medical problems. The operating room nurse combines her knowledge of surgical positions, their uses, and associated problems with her knowledge of the patient. Therefore, she ensures that the patient is optimally positioned for surgery, while being protected from adverse effects.

Surgical Positions

Position	Use
DORSAL RECUMBENT (SUPINE) The most common position and the one generally thought to be least harmful.	For any anterior approach, abdominal surgery; most extremity procedures; some thoracic procedures; head and neck surgery

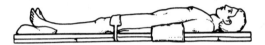

TRENDELENBURG A modification of the dorsal recumbent position	Lower abdominal surgery or when abdominal viscera need to be tilted away from the pelvic area for better exposure

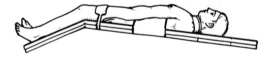

Potential Problems and Cause

CARDIOVASCULAR FUNCTION:

Possible decreased blood pressure due to decreased blood return to the heart caused by increased pressure of abdominal viscera on the inferior vena cava.

Venous thrombosis from compression of the popliteal space by a pillow or too tight leg strap

RESPIRATORY FUNCTION:

Decrease in vital capacity due to restricted posterolateral chest movement

Decrease in tidal volume

NEUROMUSCULAR FUNCTION:

Brachial plexus injury due to extension of arm more than 90 degrees

Radial (wrist drop), median (ape hand), or ulnar nerve (claw hand) damage due to arm misplacement or compression of the arm against the side of the table

Numbness on plantar surface of the foot due to tibial or sural nerve damage due to injury under the knee

INTEGUMENTARY:

Skin pressure areas

CARDIOVASCULAR FUNCTION:

Increase in blood pressure because blood pools in the upper torso; may increase intracranial pressure

RESPIRATORY FUNCTION:

14.5% decrease in vital capacity from that in sitting

A progressive decrease in tidal volume, depending upon the degree of Trendelenburg, due to decreased movement of the diaphragm because of upward displacement of abdominal viscera

Increase in intrathoracic pressure, which may decrease cardiac output

NEUROMUSCULAR FUNCTION:

Brachial plexus damage, if the shoulder braces, which are used to maintain the position with extreme angles of Trendelenburg, are misplaced over the soft tissue.

INTEGUMENTARY:

Pressure on the toes

(continued)

Surgical Positions

Position	Use
REVERSE TRENDELENBURG	Upper abdominal surgery; head and neck surgery

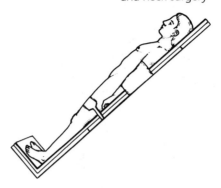

MODIFIED FOWLER'S (SITTING)	Neurosurgical procedures

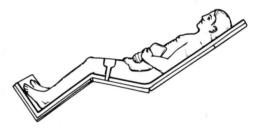

LITHOTOMY
The second most common position and the most extreme modification of the dorsal recumbent.

Perineal surgery and procedures requiring a perineal approach

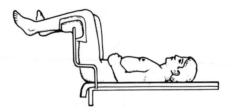

Potential Problems and Cause

CARDIOVASCULAR FUNCTION:
Decrease in mean arterial pressure

Significantly compromised circulatory system due to pooling of several hundred milliliters of blood in the lower extremities

RESPIRATORY FUNCTION:
9% decrease in vital capacity from the sitting position

CARDIOVASCULAR FUNCTION:
Hypotension due to sitting position
Development of vascular air emboli

NEUROMUSCULAR FUNCTION:
Ulnar nerve damage due to misplacement or compression of the arm against the side of the table

INTEGUMENTARY:
Development of skin pressure areas especially in ischial tuberosities due to pressure of body weight

OCULAR:
Eye injury or neck injury due to dislodgment of head holder unit

CARDIOVASCULAR FUNCTION:
Superficial thrombosis due to pressure against soft tissues of the leg by padding placed between the calves of the legs and the metal posts of the stirrups

Decrease in venous flow due to pressure of the thighs on the abdomen and abdominal viscera against the diaphragm

RESPIRATORY FUNCTION:
Decreased respiratory effectiveness due to significant restriction of diaphragmatic movement because of increased abdominal pressure from the thighs

Decrease in lung tissue compliance due to increase in pulmonary blood volume that results in engorgement of the lung tissue

18% decrease in vital capacity from sitting

Decrease in tidal volume due to extreme flexion of thighs that impairs respiratory function

(continued)

Surgical Positions

Position   Use

Lithotomy
(continued)

PRONE   Any procedure requiring a dor-
                                          sal approach

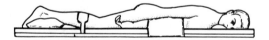

Potential Problems and Cause

NEUROMUSCULAR FUNCTION:

Pressure or crushing injury to the hand if the arms remain at the patient's sides when the end of the table is lowered or raised

Ulnar nerve damage due to pressure on the inner aspect of the elbow against the table, if the patient's arm is folded across the chest and held in place

Femoral and obturator nerve damage due to undue pressure by misplacement of instruments or leg holders

Damage to the saphenous vessels and nerves on the medial aspect of the knee due to unpadded or misplaced stirrups

Peroneal nerve damage on the lateral aspect of the knee due to unpadded or misplaced stirrups

Sciatic nerve damage is common when the legs are not raised and lowered together

CARDIOVASCULAR FUNCTION:

Decrease in blood pressure

Compromised venous return due to a tight leg restraint, dependent lower extremities, and visceral compression of the inferior vena cava

RESPIRATORY FUNCTION:

Decreased respiratory function due to restriction of normal antero-lateral respiratory movement and inhibition of normal diaphragmatic movement due to compressed abdominal wall

NEUROMUSCULAR:

Compression of the radial nerve against the humerus if the forearm hangs over the side of the table

Overextension of shoulders unless elbows are flexed and palms pronated

INTEGUMENTARY:

Pressure on the toes due to improper support of the feet and legs

Pressure on the ear, eye, superficial nerves, and blood vessels of the face due to misplaced or insufficient padding

Skin pressure areas on the chest, knees, ankles, shoulders, and iliac crest in thin individuals due to inadequate padding

(continued)

Surgical Positions

Position	Use
JACKKNIFE OR KRASKE	
A modification of the prone position	Proctological procedures

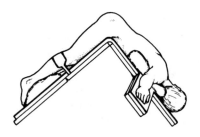

LATERAL	Upper ureter, hip, thoracic, or kidney procedures

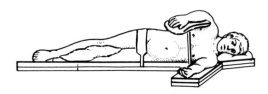

LATERAL CHEST	Approach to the uppermost thoracic cavity
LATERAL KIDNEY	Approach to the retroperitoneal space of the flank

Potential Problems and Cause

CARDIOVASCULAR FUNCTION:

Significant drop in mean arterial pressure due to pooling of blood in the chest and feet

Decrease in venous return due to dependent pooling and mechanical obstruction (at the point of the table break) and due to decreased negative intrathoracic pressure

Decrease in cardiac output due to slowed venous return, and obtundation of compensatory mechanisms by anesthesia

RESPIRATORY FUNCTION:

Decreased vital capacity by 12.5% due to restricted diaphragmatic movement and to increased blood volume in the lungs

Decreased lung compliance due to increased blood volume in the lungs

INTEGUMENTARY:

Skin pressure areas on chest, knees, ankles, and shoulders and iliac crests in thin individuals, also on the pubis at the table break due to lack of padding

CARDIOVASCULAR FUNCTION:

Decrease in systolic and diastolic pressures

Compromised circulation due to blood pooling in the lower limbs

RESPIRATORY FUNCTION:

Reduction in vital capacity and tidal volume due to weight of body on the lower chest

Reduction in diaphragmatic movement due to flexion of lower legs toward the abdomen

NEUROMUSCULAR FUNCTION:

Damage to the brachial plexus and the median, radial, and ulnar nerves due to improper support of the upper arm

Peroneal nerve damage due to compression of the down knee against a hard surface

CARDIOVASCULAR FUNCTION:

Kidney rest can markedly decrease venous return

Bibliography

Association of Operating Room Nurses, Inc: AORN Standards and Recommended Practices for Perioperative Nursing. Denver, The Association of Operating Room Nurses, 1983

Foster CG, Mukai G, Breckenridge FJ, Smith CM: Effects of surgical positioning. AORN 30(2): 219–232, August 1979

Groah LK: Operating Room Nursing–The Perioperative Role. Reston, VA, Reston Publishing, 1983

Gruendemann BJ, Meeker MH: Alexander's Care of the Patient in Surgery, 7th ed. St. Louis, CV Mosby, 1983

Julian R: Understanding Anesthesia. Menlo Park, CA, Addison–Wesley, 1984

Kim MJ, McFarland GK, McLane AM (eds): Pocket Guide to Nursing Diagnoses. St. Louis, CV Mosby, 1984

Kneedler JA, Dodge G: Perioperative Patient Care. Boston, Blackwell Scientific Publications, 1983

Meckes PF: Perioperative care of the elderly patient. Today's OR Nurse 6(9): 8–15, September 1984

Ng L, McCormick KA: Position changes and their physiological consequences. Adv Nurs Sci 4(4): 13–25, July 1982

Yoder ME: Nursing diagnosis: Applications in perioperative practice. AORN 40(2): 183–188, August 1984

5 | Anesthesia and Its Adjuncts

The duty of the anesthetist towards his patient is to take care.

While anesthetized, the patient is dependent upon the operating room nurse, anesthesiologist, and surgeon for his well-being. Although the anesthesiologist is ultimately responsible for delivering anesthesia safely, the circulating nurse maintains contact with the patient during induction and provides psychological support. Knowledge of anesthetic agents, adjuncts to anesthetic agents, and techniques that facilitate anesthesia helps the nurse protect the patient from injury.

| Anesthetic Agents

Anesthetic agents are central nervous system depressants. They have an affinity for nervous tissue, and their action reverses when they are eliminated from the cells.

The two major classifications of anesthetic agents are general and regional. The former produces narcosis (stupor or loss of consciousness) and general loss of sensation. Analgesia precedes the loss of consciousness, and varying degrees of muscular relaxation accompany it. Regional anesthetic agents do not produce loss of consciousness. However, when applied locally to any type of nerve tissue in any part of the nervous system, they block nerve conduction and thus abolish nerve sensation. The two types of anesthetic agents are compared below.

Major Classifications of Anesthetic Agents

Classification	Action	Routes of Administration	Effects
General	Blocks central awareness centers	Inhalation; intravenous; rectal; oral	Loss of consciousness; general loss of sensation; skeletal muscle relaxation; reduction of reflexes
Regional	Blocks transmission of all nerve impulses along nerve	Injection; nerve infiltration; extradural; spinal	Nerve sensation abolished over a specific body area
	Blocks transmission of nerve impulses at site of origin	Topical; local infiltration	Nerve sensation abolished over a limited body area

General Anesthesia

General anesthesia is a drug-induced state. Drugs alter the central nervous system to produce varying degrees of analgesia, depression of consciousness, skeletal muscle relaxation, and reflex reduction in the body. Although general anesthetic agents may be administered rectally, orally, or intravenously, they are most comonly administered via inhalation. An advantage of the inhalation agents is that they are excreted rapidly, and their effects are reversible more quickly than those of nonvolatile drugs administered by other routes.

General anesthesia has both advantages and disadvantages. Advantages include the facts that it is highly flexible and can be used for any surgery, for a patient of any age, and for any anatomical problem. Regardless of the operating time, the patient remains comfortable and unaware of stimuli. Disadvantages are associated with circulatory and respiratory depression. The latter is implicated in many deaths attributed to general anesthesia.

Stages of General Anesthesia

There are four stages of anesthesia. However, not all stages are seen with all anesthetics, and the stages vary with the anesthetic, the speed of induction, and the skill of the anesthetist. The early stages of anesthesia may not be seen because anesthesia is usually induced with an intravenously administered medication prior to inhalation. This facilitates the rapid transition from consciousness to surgical anesthesia. Table 5-1 identifies the four stages of anesthesia, the duration of each stage, and the patient's status in each stage, and Figure 5-1 illustrates the levels of disappearance of reflexes.

Balanced Anesthesia

In balanced or combination anesthesia, two or more drugs are combined to produce the desired general anesthetic effect. For example, neuroleptanesthesia is a form of balanced anesthesia in which nitrous oxide, oxygen, droperidol, fentanyl, and muscle relaxants are given. Advantages of balanced anesthesia include rapid induction, minimal cardiac depression, minor effects on cardiac output and smooth muscle tone, and minimal adverse effects such as postoperative nausea, excitement, and pain.

Balanced anesthesia not only produces sleep and analgesia, but also eliminates certain reflexes and provides good muscle relaxation. These goals are achieved using the following:

1. Premedication with a barbiturate, a narcotic analgesic (meperidine, morphine, fentanyl), and a parasympathetic inhibitor (atropine).
2. Induction with an intravenous or ultra short-acting barbiturate anesthetic (thiopental). Other drugs used for induction include narcotics, ketamine, and nitrous oxide plus halothane.
3. Maintenance of general anesthesia with an anesthetic gas (nitrous oxide), possibly in conjunction with an intravenous barbiturate or narcotic analgesic (meperidine, morphine, fentanyl, or Sufentanil, a newly released drug reported to be 600 times as potent as morphine).
4. Maintenance of muscle relaxation with a curare-type drug as a neuromuscular blocking agent with controlled ventilation.[1] Table 5-2 identifies the contribution by pharmacologic agents to each of the three components of the state of general anesthesia. Factors affecting drug choice, dose, and frequency include the patient's physical and emotional status; his age and drug history; the procedure to be performed, including its length; the surgeon's requirements, and the preference of the anesthesiologist.

General Anesthetics

General anesthetics are usually divided into two groups: inhalation agents and intravenous agents. Inhalation agents include gases, nonhalogenated volatile liquids, and halogenated volatile liquids. Intravenous agents include barbiturates, nonbarbiturates, and opiates. Most intravenous anesthetics are opiates.

Inhalation or volatile agents are gases, such as nitrous oxide or liquids, such as halothane. When mixed with oxygen and administered by inhalation these agents reach a concentration in the blood and brain that depresses the

Table 5-1
Stages of Anesthesia*

Stage	Duration	Patient Status
I — Analgesia**	From the administration of an anesthetic to the beginning of loss of consciousness	The sense of smell and the feeling of pain are abolished before the patient loses consciousness.
		The patient may experience vivid dreams and auditory or visual hallucinations.
		The patient's speech becomes difficult and indistinct.
		Numbness gradually spreads over the body, which feels stiff and unmanageable.
II — Excitement or Delirium**	From loss of consciousness to the loss of eyelid reflexes	The reflexes are still present, but may be exaggerated.
		The patient is particularly susceptible to external stimuli.
		Due to an increase in autonomic activity, the patient may breathe rapidly and irregularly.
		Phonation, gross motor activity, and emesis may all occur.
III — Surgical Anesthesia	From the loss of eyelid reflexes to cessation of respiratory effort	Respirations become full and regular.
	Plane 1. From beginning of automatic respiration to cessation of eyeball movement.	The eyeballs gradually move less and then cease to move.
	Plane 2. From cessation of eyeball movement to beginning of intercostal paralysis.	The pupils of the eyes constrict to the size they are in natural sleep and react sluggishly to light.
	Plane 3. From beginning to completion of intercostal paralysis.	The face is calm and expressionless and may be flushed or cyanotic.
	Plane 4. From complete intercostal paralysis to diaphragmatic paralysis.	The musculature becomes increasingly relaxed.
	NOTE: Recently there has been a tendency to divide surgical anesthesia into three planes:	The body temperature drops.
	1. Light Anesthesia: Until the eyeballs become fixed.	The pulse remains full and strong.
		The blood pressure may be slightly lowered.

Table 5-1 (Continued)
Stages of Anesthesia*

Stage	Duration	Patient Status
	2. Medium Anesthesia: Increasing intercostal paralysis. 3. Deep Anesthesia: Diaphragmatic respiration.	
IV—Overdosage or Medullary Paralysis	From onset of diaphragmatic paralysis to apnea and death	Respiratory arrest precedes vasomotor collapse. Death will occur unless the anesthetic is discontinued immediately, counteracting drugs are given, and artificial respiration performed.

*Using Volatile Agents (especially ether)
**Stages 1 and 2 are called The Stage of Induction

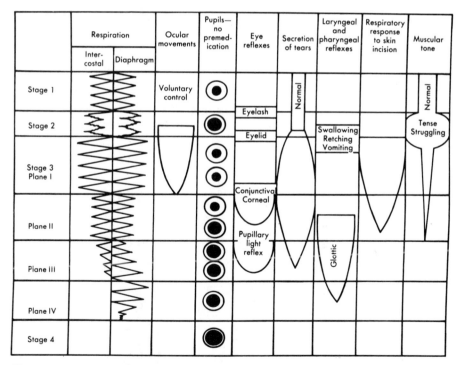

Figure 5-1. Changes occurring during anesthesia as seen with ether anesthesia. The actions of different anesthetics vary slightly from this. (After Guedel; from Atkinson RS, Rushman GB, Lee JA: A synopsis of anaesthesia. London, John Wright & Sons, 1982)

Table 5-2
The Contribution by Pharmacologic Agents to Each of the Three Components of the State of General Anesthesia

	Barbiturates	Etomidate	Opiates	Nitrous Oxide	Halothane	Enflurane	Isoflurane	Ketamine	Benzodiazepines	Succinylcholine	Non-depolarizing Neuro-Muscular Blockers
Amnesia and unconsciousness	4	4	1–2	2	4	4	4	4	2–3	0	0
Analgesia	0	0	3–4	2	4	4	4	3	0	0	0
Muscle relaxation	0	0	0	0	1–2	2–3	2–3	0	0	4	4

The number 0 to 4 in the above table refers to the relative intensity of effect induced by each agent, with 0 indicating no effect and 4 the greatest effect. (From Julien R: Understanding Anesthesia, p. 152. Menlo Park, CA. Addison–Wesley. 1984) central nervous system and causes anesthesia or narcosis. Table 5-3 identifies some of these agents, their uses, advantages, disadvantages, contraindications, and postoperative nursing implications.

Regional Anesthesia

Regional anesthesia can be achieved by depositing the appropriate drug on or near the nerve or nerve pathway anywhere between the site of the painful stimuli and the central nervous system receptors. Therefore, because the anesthetic affects only a specific area and not cortical functions, the patient remains awake throughout the entire procedure and has control of his airway. Additionally, respiration is spontaneous. Regional anesthetics are used for diagnostic procedures, treatments, examinations, and surgery.

Drugs used to produce regional anesthesia can be applied topically or injected. Table 5-4 identifies six categories of regional anesthesia techniques and their major uses. Table 5-5 describes the properties of commonly used regional anesthetics.

Surface (Topical) Anesthetic

Surface anesthetics are used on mucous membranes, damaged skin surfaces, wounds, and burns. They do not penetrate unbroken skin. Local anesthetics, in the form of solutions, ointments, gels, creams, or powders, produce loss of sensation by paralyzing afferent nerve endings. Topical anesthesia is used for surgical procedures on the nose and throat to eliminate pharyngeal and tracheal reflexes during bronchoscopy. In addition, it is used in such genitourinary procedures as urethral meatotomy and cystoscopy. Cocaine in a 4% to 10% solution is one of the most widely used agents for topical anesthesia.

Local Infiltration

Local infiltration is achieved by injecting dilute solutions (0.1%) of the drug into the area to be incised. The anesthetic blocks the subcutaneous branches of sensory nerves, thus producing sensory blockade of nerve endings in the skin. Local anesthesia is used for such minor procedures as incision and drainage of an abscess, removal of small tumors, suturing of wounds, and thoracentesis.

Epinephrine (1 : 100,000 or 1 : 2000,000) is often added to the solution. The vasoconstrictor effect of the epinephrine intensifies and prolongs the anesthesia in a limited region. Additionally, it prevents excessive bleeding and delays vascular absorption of the local anesthetic, thereby decreasing systemic effects. Epinephrine should never be added to solutions in blocks of toes, fingers, or the penis because the ischemia can result in gangrene.

Conduction Block

In conduction block, a local anesthetic is injected around nerve trunks that supply the surgical site. A conduction block can be performed on most major nerves, for example, the brachial plexus, branches of the trigeminal nerve, and

Table 5-3
General Anesthetics

Agent	Use	Advantages	Disadvantages	Contraindications	Postoperative Nursing Implications
Inhalation Agents					
Gases: Nitrous oxide	Maintenance; occasionally for induction; brief induction	Has little effect on heart rate, myocardial contractility, respiration, blood pressure, liver, kidneys or metabolism in absence of hypoxia	Requires low oxygen concentration for the surgical level of anesthesia		Monitor for signs of hypoxemia
		Produces excellent analgesia	Possible hypoxemia with excessive amounts		
		Rapid induction and emergence	Weak anesthetic		
		Does not result in increased capillary bleeding	No muscular relaxation; a neuromuscular blocking agent must be used in procedures requiring muscular relaxation		
		Does not sensitize the myocardium to epinephrine			
		Nonemetic			
		Nonflammable; nonexplosive			
Halogenated Volatile Liquids:					
Halothane (Fluothane)	Maintenance; commonly used for pediatric inhalational induction	Easy to administer	Myocardial depressant	Most obstetric deliveries except in very low concentrations	Watch for dysrhythmias, hypotension, respiratory depression
		Rapid, smooth induction and recovery	Can cause dysrhythmias		

122

Agent	Use	Advantages	Disadvantages	Precautions	Nursing considerations
		Has a relatively pleasant odor; nonirritating; Depresses salivary and bronchial secretions; Potent bronchodilator; Easily suppresses pharyngeal and laryngeal reflexes; Nonflammable and nonexplosive	Sensitizes the heart to action of catecholamine; Circulatory-respiratory depression is dose dependent; Has no analgesic property; Shivering with emergence	Patients with known hepatic or biliary disease or markedly increased intracranial pressure	Body temperature may fall and patient may shiver following prolonged use; Shivering increases oxygen consumption
Enflurane (Ethrane)	Maintenance; occasionally for induction	Pleasant; Rapid induction and recovery; Nonirritating, no secretions; Bronchodilator; Good muscle relaxant; Cardiac rhythm very stable; Nonemetic; Nonflammable and nonexplosive	Myocardial depressant; As depth of anesthesia increases, so does hypotension; Shivering with emergence	Use cautiously in patients with renal disease	Monitor patient for decreased heart and respiratory rates and hypotension; Shivering increases oxygen consumption
Isoflurane (Forane)	Maintenance; occasionally for induction	Rapid induction and recovery; Bronchodilator	Circulatory-respiratory depression is dose dependent	Avoid use in patients with impaired renal function	Watch for respiratory depression; hypotension

(continued)

Table 5-3 (Continued)
General Anesthetics

Agent	Use	Advantages	Disadvantages	Contraindications	Postoperative Nursing Implications
Isoflurane (continued)		Excellent muscle relaxant	Potentiates the action of nondepolarizing muscular relaxants		Shivering increases oxygen consumption
		Extremely stable cardiac rhythm	May shiver		
		Compatible with epinephrine	Blood pressure tends to drop as depth of anesthesia increases, but pulse remains somewhat elevated		
		Nonflammable and nonexplosive			
Intravenous Agents:					
Barbiturates Thiopental sodium (Pentothal sodium); thiopentone	Primary use is induction of general anesthesia	Rapid, smooth and plesant induction; quick recovery	Associated with hypoxemia, airway obstruction, and respiratory depression	Contraindicated for use in patients with severe cardiac failure, peripheral circulatory collapse, severe uremia, compromised airway, status asthmaticus, latent or manifest porphyria and in those with a known hypersensitivity to barbiturates	Watch for signs and symptoms of hypoxemia, airway obstruction, and cardiovascular and respiratory depression
		Infrequent complications	No muscle relaxation		
		No secretions	Little analgesia		
		Nonemetic	Has a tendency to produce laryngospasm		
		No sensitization of autonomic tissues of heart to catecholamines	Cardiovascular depression, especially in hypovolemic or debilitated patients		
		Nonexplosive			

Drug					
Benzodiazepines					
Diazepam (Valium)	Induction of general anesthesia; provides amnesia during balanced anesthesia	Minimally affects the cardiovascular system Causes little respiratory depression Is a potent anticonvulsant	Irritating when injected into a peripheral vein Has a long elimination half-life Poor analgesia and relaxation Phlebitis	Prohibited in patients with absence of veins suitable for intravenous administration because extravascular infiltration leads to sloughing and tissue necrosis	Monitor patient's vital signs
Nonbarbiturates					
Ketamine hydrochloride (Ketalar, Ketaject)	Produces a dissociative state of consciousness. Induction when a barbiturate is contraindicated. Sole anesthetic agent for short diagnostic and surgical procedures not requiring skeletal muscle relaxation, especially in children	Produces rapid anesthesia and profound analgesia Solution is not irritating to veins or tissues Because laryngeal and pharyngeal reflexes may be obtunded, patent airway can be maintained without endotracheal intubation Muscle tone is preserved	Emergence may be accompanied by unpleasant dreams, hallucinations and emergence delirium Increases heart rate, blood pressure, and intraocular pressure Poor relaxation	Contraindicated for patients with a history of increased cerebrospinal pressure, cardiovascular accident, psychiatric problems, and with hypertension Contraindicated for intraocular surgery	Protect patient from visual, tactile, and auditory stimuli during recovery Monitor patient's vital signs

(continued)

Table 5-3 (Continued)
General Anesthetics

Agent	Use	Advantages	Disadvantages	Contraindications	Postoperative Nursing Implications
Nonbarbiturates					
Etomidate (Amidate)	Induction. Indicated in high risk patients with low cardiac reserves, patients allergic to barbiturates, and possibly in trauma patients, including those with increased intracranial pressure	Rapid induction Has less cardiac and respiratory depressant effects than thiopental	Causes muscle fasciculations and pain on injection Causes emergence reactions and nausea and vomiting Lack of analgesia	Not approved for use in children less than 10 years of age and pregnant women	Watch for nausea and vomiting. Protect patient from visual, tactile, and auditory stimuli during recovery Observe injection site for phlebitis
Tranquilizers					
Droperidol (Inapsine)	Used preoperatively and during induction and maintenance of anesthesia as an adjunct to general or regional anesthesia	Rapid, smooth induction and recovery Produces sleepiness and mental detachment for several hours Is an antiemetic	May cause hypotension because it is a peripheral vasodilator	Use with caution in elderly or debilitated patients, in those who have received depressant drugs, and in those with cardiovascular disease	Monitor patient for increased pulse rate and hypotension
Narcotics					
Fentanyl citrate (Sublimaze)	Used preoperatively for minor and major surgery, urologic procedures, and gastroscopy As an adjunct to regional anesthesia,	Rapid, smooth induction and recovery Does not release histamine Minimally affects the cardiovascular system	Side effects include respiratory depression, euphoria, bradycardia, bronchoconstriction, nausea, vomiting, and miosis	Contraindicated in patients who have received MAO inhibitors within 14 days and who have myasthenia gravis Use cautiously in patients with head	Observe for respiratory depression Watch for nausea and vomiting and position to prevent aspiration, if vomiting occurs Monitor blood pressure

	induction and maintenance of general anesthesia	Reversible with a narcotic antagonist (naloxone)		injuries, respiratory depression, and in patients who are hypovolemic, debilitated, and/or elderly	Decrease postoperative narcotics to 1/3 to 1/4 usual dose
Neuroleptics Droperidol and fentanyl (Innovar)	Used for short procedures in which a conscious patient is required	Rapid, smooth induction and recovery	Causes respiratory depression, extrapyramidal symptoms, apnea, laryngospasm, bronchospasm, bradycardia, and hallucinations	Use cautiously in children, in patients with impaired liver, kidney, or pulmonary function and in those who are poor surgical risks	Closely monitor patient's vital signs
	Used as a premedication and as an adjunct for induction and maintenance of general anesthesia	Somnolence without total unconsciousness		Contraindicated in patients with parkinsonism and in patients who have taken MAO inhibitor therapy within the past 14 days	
		Psychological indifference to the environment			
		No voluntary movements			
		Less analgesia required postoperatively			
		Satisfactory amnesia			

Table 5-4
Regional Anesthesia Techniques

Technique	Use(s)
Surface (topical) anesthetic	Sensory block of mucous membranes
Local infiltration	Block of subcutaneous branches of sensory nerves
Conduction (nerve) block	Motor and sensory block by interrupting nerve conduction
Intravenous (Bier) block	Sensory block of upper and lower extremities
Peridural (epidural, caudal) block	Motor, sensory, and autonomic block of nerve roots and spinal cord
Subdural (spinal, saddle) block	Motor, sensory, and autonomic block of nerve roots and spinal cord

From Julien R: Understanding Anesthesia, p 163. Menlo Park, CA, Addison–Wesley, 1984

the femoral or sciatic nerves. These blocks allow surgery on the arm and hand, teeth, jaws, and face, and leg and foot, respectively.

Intravenous (Bier) Block

This intravenous regional technique is used to produce anesthesia below the elbow or knee. After a pneumatic tourniquet has been applied to cut off arterial blood flow, a local anesthetic is injected into the vein of the limb to be anesthetized. The anesthetic fills the collapsed veins, and the tourniquet prevents its systemic dissemination.

Peridural Block

This block necessitates injection into the spinal cord. Injection of an anesthetic into the peridural sheath is referred to as a peridural anesthesia. The motor, sensory, and autonomic neruons in the nerve roots in contact with the solution are blocked.

Peridural anesthesia can be one of two types, epidural or caudal, depending upon the route of entry into the spinal cord. Additionally, each technique allows either a single or continuous dose of anesthetic to be administered.

Subdural Block

Spinal anesthesia is a type of extensive conduction nerve block in which a local anesthetic is injected into the subarachnoid space. This causes motor, sensory, and autonomic blockade of those nerve roots in contact with the solution. Spinal anesthesia is used for surgery of the lower extremities, perineum, lower abdomen, and inguinal area.

Usually, the patient is placed in the lateral position, and the drug, in a solution with a specific gravity greater than that of spinal fluid (a hyperbaric solution), is injected. After the needle is withdrawn, the patient is turned supine. A hyperbaric solution tends to diffuse downward, and dose and patient position determine the level of the block. For example, placing the

Table 5-5
Properties of Commonly Used Regional Anesthetics

	Cocaine	Procaine	Benzocaine	Lidocaine	Tetracaine	Mepivacaine	Bupivacaine
Trade Names	—	Novocain	Americaine Hurricane	Xylocaine Lignocaine	Pontocaine	Carbocaine	Marcaine
Potency	2 to 3 times that of procaine		Very low	2 times that of procaine	10 times that of procaine	2 times that of procaine	
Onset of Action	1 minute	2 to 5 minutes	Immediate	Immediate	5 to 10 minutes	Less rapid than procaine	5 to 15 minutes
Duration of Action	1 hour	1 hour	During contact only	1 to 2 hours	1-1/2 to 2 hours	More prolonged (2–4 hours) than procaine or lidocaine	180 to 600 minutes
Dose	1% to 4% topically 5% to 10% for anesthesia of nose and throat	0.25% to 2%, depending upon method of administration 10% for spinal anesthesia Not used topically	Variable; 5% to 10% ointment topically	0.5% to 4% for injection 2% and 5% topically	0.5% to 2% topically 0.15% to 0.25% for injection	1% to 2% solution	0.25% to 0.75% for injection
Toxicity	4 times more toxic than procaine when injected subcutaneously; toxic dose is 300 mg — this is easily reached with 3cc of 10% solution	Least toxic of all local anesthetics	Relatively nontoxic	Like that of procaine	More toxic than procaine, but toxic effects rare because of low dosage used	2 times that of procaine — less than lidocaine	Like other local anesthetics, as potency increases so does potential for toxicity Like others, large IV doses or blood levels result in CNS toxicity—seizures, respiratory arrest, and cardiovascular collapse

(continued)

129

Table 5-5 (Continued)
Properties of Commonly Used Regional Anesthetics

	Cocaine	Procaine	Benzocaine	Lidocaine	Tetracaine	Mepivacaine	Bupivacaine
Precautions	Not recommended for infiltration, nerve block, or spinal anesthesia Repeated use causes psychic dependence Repeated use in eye may cause clouding, pitting, ulceration of cornea, and mydriasis	Over-dose or rapid injection may cause stimulation	Suitable for topical use only Sensitization may develop Sprays are not dose-metered and excess amounts easily given	When administered rapidly or in large doses may cause convulsions and hypotension	May cause vasodepressor effects		

Adapted from Hahn AB, Barkin RL, Oestreich SKJ: Pharmacology in Nursing, 15th ed, p 256–257. St. Louis, CV Mosby, 1982 patient in the Trendelenburg position moves the level of the block toward the chest. Sometimes a hypobaric solution, that is, one with a specific gravity less than that of spinal fluid, is used. A solution with a specific gravity less than that of spinal fluid tends to diffuse upward, and so the patient is positioned with the operative site uppermost (for example, the jackknife position for a hemorrhoidectomy).

Onset of anesthesia occurs within 1 to 2 minutes after injection and lasts 60 to 180 minutes, depending upon the dose and type of anesthetic. The patient does not experience pain during the procedure but may be aware of pulling sensations. These sensations may cause feelings of faintness and nausea. Side-effects of spinal anesthesia include marked hypotension, postspinal headache, urinary retention, and high spinal blockage, with paralysis of intercostal muscles, bradycardia and unconsciousness.

| Neuromuscular Blocking Agents

Neuromuscular blocking agents are important muscle relaxants and are used as adjuncts to anesthesia for two reasons. One, they produce adequate muscle relaxation during anesthesia and decrease the amount of general anesthetic needed. And two, they facilitate endotracheal intubation and prevent laryngospasm. However, neuromuscular blocking agents do not affect pain or other sensory perception. Although these drugs may be given intramuscularly, the intravenous route is preferred because onset of action is faster and more predictable.

Common to all neuromuscular blocking agents postoperatively is the potential for residual muscle weakness, if reversal is incomplete or renal inefficiency is present. This may manifest as inadequate respiratory function, with hypoventilation and hypoxemia/hypercarbia. Other acute side-effects common to many neuromuscular blocking agents include hypotension, bronchospasm, and cardiac disturbances. Sympathetic ganglionic blockade and histamine release, both of which cause peripheral vasodilation, are believed to cause hypotension. The release of histamine is also thought to cause bronchospasm. However, the degree of histamine released varies considerably with different muscle relaxants.

Neuromuscular blocking agents are classified as nondepolarizing, or competitive, and depolarizing. Nondepolarizing agents (also called curariform) such as tubocurarine, metocurine, gallamine, pancuronium bromide, atracurium besylate, and vecuronium bromide, have a slower onset than depolarizing agents such a succinylcholine chloride. In addition, with the exception of atracurium besylate and vecuronium bromide, nondepolarizing agents have a significantly longer duration of action than depolarizing agents.

Nondepolarizing Neuromuscular Blocking Agents

Nondepolarizing or competitive neuromuscular blocking agents occupy the cholinergic receptor sites at the myoneural junction and produce skeletal muscle relaxation. By preventing acetylcholine from acting on these sites, nondepolarizing blocking agents prevent depolarization of the postsynaptic membrane. Therefore, the muscle fibers are not stimulated and skeletal muscle cannot contract. The mechanism of action of these drugs involves alterations in the movement of potassium and sodium ions that are responsible for the depolarization and the repolarization of the muscle membranes.

Anticholinesterases such as neostigmine, pyridostigmine, and edrophonium, increase acetylcholine concentration at the motor end-plate. These drugs are used to reverse nondepolarizing neuromuscular blockade. Administration of anticholinesterases is preceded by an intravenous injection of atropine that antagonizes undesired muscarinic actions of acetylcholine such as bradycardia and increased salivation. The effects of neostigmine last for one half to one and a half hours. The effects of small doses of edrophonium last up to 5 minutes, whereas in doses of 1 mg/kg, the duration of edrophonium is comparable to neostigmine. Table 5-6 lists the nondepolarizing agents, their characteristics, and their antagonists.

Depolarizing Neuromuscular Blocking Agents

Depolarizing neuromuscular blocking agents resemble acetylcholine in structure and have a high affinity for acetylcholine receptor sites. These drugs initiate depolarization of the motor end-plate at the myoneural junction. This may be observed in patients after injection of the drug as muscle fasciculations. Once the motor end-plate depolarizes, it does not repolarize and relaxation ensues. The fasciculations that precede the relaxation are believed to be the cause of postoperative muscle soreness.

Succinylcholine, a short-acting depolarizing agent, is used primarily as a single-dose injection to facilitate intubation. Table 5-7 describes its characteristics.

Induced Hypothermia

Induced hypothermia is used in most cardiac surgical procedures, particularly in pediatric cardiac surgery and cardiopulmonary bypass procedures. Defined as the deliberate reduction of body temperature for therapeutic purposes, induced hypothermia extends the period of circulatory interruption, ischemia, or hypoperfusion with minimal danger of neurologic or other organ damage. Cooling and rewarming are accomplished during cardiopulmonary bypass, via the heat exchanger of the heart-lung machine.

Induced Hypotension

Induced hypotension may be used in selected procedures to manage bleeding at the operative site. It can be used in radical head and neck surgery, pelvic exenterations, major orthopedic surgery such as disarticulation procedures, and neurosurgical procedures such as aneurysm repair. Because it decreases blood loss and minimizes oozing, induced hypotension reduces the need for transfusions. In addition, it decreases the amount of anesthetic required.

Table 5-6
Nondepolarizing Neuromuscular Blocking Agents

Agent	Onset of Action for IV Route	Duration of Action	Undesirable Action	Excretion	Antagonists	Comments
Nondepolarizing (Competitive) Blocking Agents:						
Tubocurarine chloride (Tubarine)	2 to 3 minutes	25 to 90 minutes with single large dose or multiple, single doses; may last 24 hours	Hypotension, bronchospasm	33% to 75% eliminated in urine unchanged; 10% to 20% excreted in bile	Neostigmine Edrophonium Physostigmine Pyridostigmine	Is a histamine releaser and in higher doses causes sympathetic ganglion blockade; Prolonged action in patients with renal or liver disease and in the elderly or debilitated patient
Metocurine iodide (Metubine)	3 to 5 minutes	25 to 90 minutes; 60 minutes is average; depends on the dose and general anesthetic used	Hypotension, bronchospasm	Excreted by kidney	Neostigmine Edrophonium Physostigmine Pyridostigmine	2 times as potent as curare; Weak histamine releaser (less than curare)
Gallamine (Flaxedil)	3 to 5 minutes	15 to 35 minutes	Tachycardia and hypertension; May cause allergic reaction in patients sensitive to iodine	Excreted by kidney	Neostigmine Edrophonium Physostigmine Pyridostigmine	One fifth as potent as curare; Is not chemically a curare drug but pharmacologically acts like curare; Has no effect on autonomic ganglia; Does not cause bronchospasm; Do not administer to patients with impaired renal function, will accumulate; Not the muscle relaxant of choice with cardiovascular patients

(continued)

Table 5-6 (Continued)
Nondepolarizing Neuromuscular Blocking Agents

Agent	Onset of Action for IV Route	Duration of Action	Undesirable Action	Excretion	Antagonists	Comments
Pancuronium bromide (Pavulon)	2 to 3 minutes	35 to 45 minutes	Tachycardia Transient skin rashes, and a burning sensation at injection site	Metabolized in liver; excreted by kidneys and some biliary excretion	Neostigmine Edrophonium Physostigmine Pyridostigmine	Five times more potent than curare Is a steroid derivative Does not cause ganglionic blockage and therefore does not usually cause hypotension Has a vagolytic action that increases heart rate Contraindicated in patients with history of tachycardia, in patients in whom an increase in heart rate is undesirable and in patients sensitive to bromides
Atracurium besylate (Tracrium)	2 to 3 minutes	20 to 30 minutes	Slight hypotension in a few patients	Undergoes the Hofmann elimination process (the spontaneous degredation of the molecule at physiologic pH and temperature to inactive metabolites). Does not rely on renal metabolism	Neostigmine Edrophonium Physostigmine Pyridostigmine	Qualitatively similar to pancuronium Very weak histamine releaser Minimal autonomic effects Will not accumulate with repeated doses as others do Drug of choice for patients with underlying cardiac disease Can be used in patients with hepatic and renal disease
Vecuronium bromide (Norcuron)	2 to 3 minutes	20 to 30 minutes		Probably mostly metabolized in liver (unique)	Neostigmine Edrophonium Physostigmine Pyridostigmine	Derivative of pancuronium but much shorter duration and causes less tachycardia

Table 5-7
Depolarizing Neuromuscular Blocking Agents

Agent	Onset of Action for IV Route	Duration of Action	Undesirable Action
Succinylcholine chloride (Anectine Chloride, Quelicin, Sucostrin, Sux-Cert); suxamethonium chloride	Relaxation in 1 minute; peak action in 1 to 3 minutes	5 to 10 minutes	Respiratory depression, bradycardia, salivation, hypotension, cardiac dysrhythmias, tachycardia, hypertension, cardiac arrest, and a rise in intraocular and intragastric pressure, fasciculations

Excretion	Antagonists	Comments
Most metabolized in plasma by pseudocholinesterase; 10% excreted as unchanged drug	None	Contraindicated in patients with a deficiency of plasma cholinesterase from a genetic variant defect, liver disease, uremia, or malnutrition. Use cautiously in patients with glaucoma, those having eye surgery, those with penetrating wounds of the eye, those with cardiovascular, hepatic, pulmonary, metabolic, or renal disorders. Use in patients with burns, severe trauma, spinal cord injuries, and muscle dystrophies. May result in sudden hyperkalemia and consequent cardiac arrest

Hypotension is induced pharmacologically. It can be induced by deep anesthesia with an inhalant anesthetic such as halothane or with an intravenous anesthetic that affects the vascular smooth muscle. Sodium nitroprusside is frequently used and very little of the drug is needed to produce an immediate and dramatic hypotensive state.

Induced hypotension causes various cardiac responses. Coronary perfusion remains adequate and permanent myocardial damage does not result, if the blood pressure does not fall below 60 torr. Since a prolonged state of induced hypotension can cause morbidity and mortality, vital signs are monitored frequently postoperatively. Among the most common complications are cerebral hypoxia and infarct, renal failure, oliguria and anuria, thromboembolism, persistent hypotension, and cardiac failure and arrest.

| Evaluation

The patient remains stable and free of injury throughout anesthesia.

| Summary

Although the anesthesiologist is ultimately responsible for safely administering the anesthesia, the operating nurse, with her knowledge of the patient and anesthetics and their adjuncts, ensures the patient's psychological comfort and safety.

References

1. Hahn AB, Barkin RL, Oestreich SJK: Pharmacology in Nursing, 15th ed, p 238. St. Louis, CV Mosby, 1982

Bibliography

Association of Operating Room Nurses, Inc: AORN Standards and Recommended Practices for Perioperative Nursing. Denver, The Association of Operating Room Nurses, 1983

Atkinson, RS, Rushman GB, Lee JA: A Synopsis of Anaesthesia, 9th ed. Bristol, John Wright & Sons, 1982

Clinical Anesthesia Procedures of the Massachusetts General Hospital, 2nd ed. Boston, Little, Brown & Co, 1982

Drain CB: Managing postoperative pain — It's a matter of sighs. Nurs 84 14(8): 52–55, 1984

Groah LK: Operating Room Nursing — The Perioperative Role. Reston, VA, Reston Publishing, 1983

Gruendemann BJ, Meeker MH: Alexander's Care of the Patient. In Surgery, 7th ed. St. Louis, CV Mosby, 1983

Hahn AB, Barkin RL, Oestreich SJK: Pharmacology in Nursing, 15th ed. St. Louis, CV Mosby, 1982

Julian R: Understanding Anesthesia. Menlo Park, CA, Addison-Wesley, 1984

Kneedler, JA, Dodge G: Perioperative Patient Care. Boston, Blackwell Scientific Publications, 1983

Podjasek JH: Which postop patient faces the greatest respiratory risk? RN 48(9): 44–56, 1985

Recommended practices: Monitoring the patient receiving local anesthesia. AORN 39(6): 1080–1083, May 1984

Rodman MJ, Smith DW: Clinical Pharmacology in Nursing, 2nd ed. Philadelphia, JB Lippincott, 1984

Snow J: Manual of Anesthesia, 2nd ed. Boston, Little, Brown & Co 1982

Wlody GS: Isoflurane. AORN J; 40(4): 568–571, October 1984

Yoder ME: Nursing diagnosis : Applications in perioperative practice. AORN J 40(2):183–188, August 1984

6 | Intraoperative Techniques

Medicine cannot be carried out without the basic principles of aseptic technique and wound care, the skills of handling instruments and suturing lacerations, and the techniques of access to veins, arteries, and body cavities.

—Charles W. Van Way III, Charles A. Buerk

The surgeon's knowledge and skill significantly affect the patient's intraoperative experience. However, surgery is a team effort and nurses assume one of two roles. They either circulate or scrub. The circulating nurse assists the scrub nurse and the surgeon. She helps position the patient and applies equipment and surgical drapes. She also provides the scrub nurse with supplies, disposes of equipment, and keeps a count of instruments, needles, and sponges used. The scrub nurse provides the surgeon with the correct instruments and supplies. Surgeon and nurses work together for a positive patient outcome.

Intraoperative Wound Infection Control Measures

Most infections, either endogenous or exogenous, result from contamination acquired in the operating room. Three factors primarily determine the development of a surgical wound infection. They are the microbial contamination of the wound, the condition of the wound at the end of surgery, and the susceptibility of the patient. Since the interaction of these three factors is complex, intraoperative measures intended to prevent surgical wound infection are aimed at all three. Although surgical technique during the operation determines the condition of the wound at the end of surgery, measures that prevent surgical wound infection include avoiding hair removal and cleansing the skin.

Hair Removal

One of three methods can be used to remove hair from the operative site: electric clipping, a depilatory, and shaving. However, studies have shown that different methods of hair removal are associated with varying wound infection rates. The rate of infection is considerably higher for preoperative shaving than for either no shaving or depilatory use. In one study the incidence of postoperative wound infection was 0.6% following depilatory use, but 5.6% following a razor prep.[1] In another study the infection rate was 0.9% with no skin preparation, 1.7% when hair was clipped, and 2.3 % when the standard shave was done less than 24 hours before surgery.[2]

The timing of skin preparation also affects wound infection rate when hair is removed by shaving. Shaving damages the epidermis, provides resident flora access to the operative site, and allows transient flora to penetrate the protective barrier of the skin. In one study the postoperative infection rate was 3.1% when the shave was done immediately before surgery, 7.1% when the shave was done within 24 hours of surgery, and 20% when the shave was done more than 24 hours before surgery. Thus, the longer the time between the preoperative shave and surgery, the greater the incidence of postoperative infection. The timing effect was not evident with depilatory creams.[1]

The efficiency, safety, and cost of the three methods of preoperative hair removal have also been compared. The safety razor produced both gross cuts and epidermal damage. The electric clippers caused nips and cuts at skin creases. And although the depilatory caused no skin damage, lymphocytic infiltration was observed on histologic examination of skin biopsy specimens taken 24 hours after its application.[3]

The Centers for Disease Control recommends that hair near the operative site not be removed unless it will interfere with the surgical procedure. Additionally, if hair removal is necessary, clipping or the use of a depilatory is advocated. Similarly, the Association of Operating Room Nurses recommends that hair be removed from the operative site only as necessary. Furthermore, if hair is to be removed by shaving, the razor must be sharp, well-designed, and either disposable or terminally sterilized. A wet shave is preferable and should be done as near the operative time as possible. Preoperative hair removal should be done by a person with demonstrated skill and efficiency in the procedure.

Skin Cleansing and Disinfection

The skin around the operative site is thoroughly cleansed before surgery to remove superficial flora, soil, and debris. This reduces the risk of the patient's skin flora contaminating the wound. Just before surgery, a preoperative skin preparation is applied to kill or minimize the deeper resident flora. Factors considered in skin disinfection include the condition of the area; the number and kinds of contaminants; the characteristics of the skin to be disinfected, and the patient's general physical condition.

Once the patient has been properly positioned on the operating room table and anesthetized, a scrubbed member of the surgical team completes the final skin cleansing and disinfection. If the patient has not showered just before coming to the operating room, the surgical site is scrubbed with an antimicrobial scrub solution and disinfected with an antimicrobial solution.

Some physicians prefer that the operative site be *painted* rather than scrubbed. This may be desirable when vigorous pressure and friction would disseminate a condition. For example, malignant cells could be freed into the blood and lymph streams or a plaque in a carotid artery could be dislodged.

The site of the incision and the nature of the surgery determine the extent of the area to be prepared. Figure 6-1 illustrates areas to be prepared for various procedures.

Patient Draping

The purpose of draping is to establish a sterile field around the operative site, thus preventing the passage of microorganisms between nonsterile and sterile areas. The incision site is the only area exposed. Sterile drapes cover all unprepared areas of the patient. Whether single-use or reusable, surgical drapes should be resistant to blood and liquid penetration.

Although their use is controversial and depends upon physician preference, plastic incisional drapes are sometimes used as an adjunct to conventional drapes. When applied after the fabric drape, they obviate the need for towel clamps.

When used alone incisional drapes form a complete seal over the skin, thus protecting the wound from bacteria and excretions. Skin color and anatomical landmarks are easily visible and the incision is made through the drape.

Plastic incisional drapes are alleged to have both advantages and disadvantages, and studies support both views. For example, plastic incisional drapes have been found to inhibit the migration of microorganisms and to isolate gross sources of contamination. Conversely, bacterial growth has been found to increase at the edges of plastic incisional drapes, if improperly used.

Incisions

Factors that determine the location of a surgical incision include the diagnosis of the patient's condition and the pathology that the surgeon expects to find. The incision must allow adequate exposure, be minimally traumatizing, cosmetically effective, easily extended, easily closed, cause minimal postoperative discomfort, and offer maximal postoperative wound strength. In surgical emergencies, the incision must also offer rapid and easy entry. Table 6-1 illustrates some common surgical incisions and describes these incisions, including location, characteristics, and uses.

Preoperative Preparation of the Patient

Thyroid prep. Extends from chinline to nipples, including axillary region. Extend to back of neck and upper shoulder, as sketched.

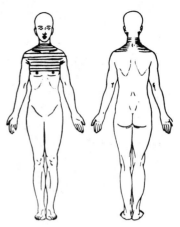

Parathyroid prep (as for sternal splitting). Extends from chinline to umbilicus, shoulder to shoulder in the front. Extend to back of neck and upper shoulder in back, as shown. Prep laterally for chest tubes if so ordered.

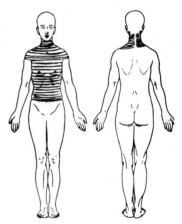

Thoracotomy prep. Extends from chinline to iliac crest, from nipple on unaffected side to at least 2 inches beyond the midline in back. Include axilla and entire arm to elbow.

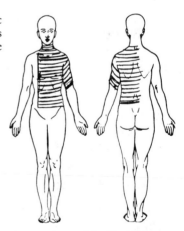

Figure 6-1. Areas of skin to be prepared for surgical procedures. (Modified from Walter CW: In Current Practice Bulletin No. 7-2-5. Boston, Peter Bent Brigham Hospital, March, 1975. Redrawn for Altemeier WA, Burke JF, Pruitt Jr, BA, Sandusky WR by American College of Surgeons: Manual on Control of Infection in Surgical Patients, 2nd ed, Charlottesville, VA, 1984)

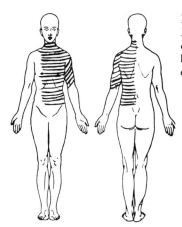

Preoperative Preparation of the Patient
Mastectomy prep. Extends from upper neck to iliac crest, from nippleline on unaffected side to midline of back (affected side). Prep axilla and entire arm to elbow on affected side.

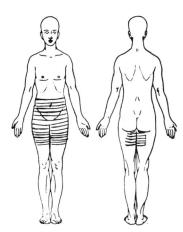

Lower abdominal prep (as for hernia, femoral vein ligation, femoral embolectomy). Extends from 2 inches above the umbilicus to mid-thigh, including the pubic area. Femoral ligation — preparation area to midline of thigh posteriorly. Hernia and embolectomy — prepare to costal margin and down to knee, as ordered.

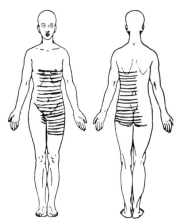

Flank prep (as for renal procedures, adrenalectomy, sympathectomy). Extends from nippleline to pubis and 3 inches beyond the midline in back. Prepare pubic area. Prepare upper thigh on the affected side.

Preoperative Preparation of the Patient
Abdominal prep. Extends from 3 inches above the nippleline to upper thighs, including pubis.

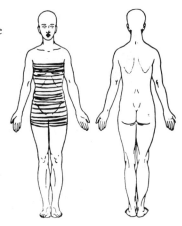

Perineal prep (as for hemorrhoidectomy, fistula-inano, pilonidal sinus). Extends from pubis, perineum, and perianal area, from the waist in back to at least 3 inches below the groin.

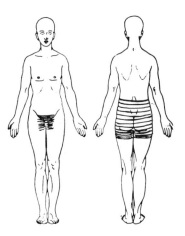

Spine prep. Extends from entire back including shoulders and neck to hairline and down to knees and to both sides, including axillae.

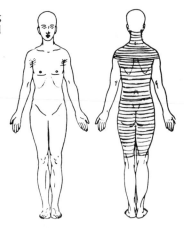

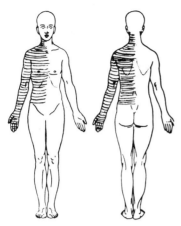

Preoperative Preparation of the Patient
Shoulder prep. Extends from fingertips to hairline, midline chest to midline spine on operative side and to iliac crest, including axillae.

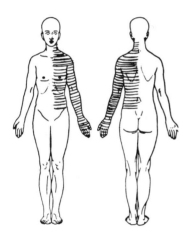

Upper arm prep. Extends from fingertips to neckline (hairline), on operative side from midline chest to midline spine, on operative side from axilla to iliac crest. Trim and clean fingernails. Use brush on hand and nails.

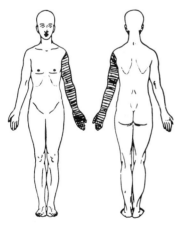

Hand prep. Extends from fingertips to shoulder. Trim and clean fingernails. Use brush on hand and nails.

Preoperative Preparation of the Patient
Forearm and elbow prep. Extends from fingernails to shoulder, including axilla. Trim and clean fingernails. Use brush on hand and nails.

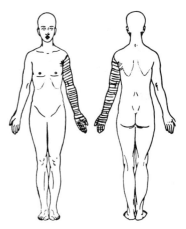

Saphenous vein ligation prep. Extends from umbilicus to toes of affected leg, or both legs. Include pubis and perineal area. Prep entire leg posteriorly.

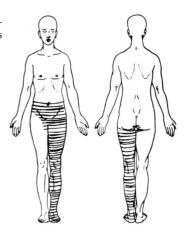

Thigh prep. Extends from toes to 3 inches above the umbilicus, midline front and back, including complete pubic area. Clean and trim toenails. Use brush on foot and nails.

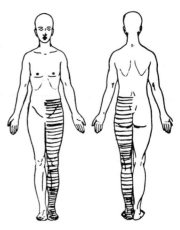

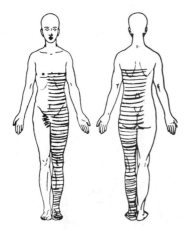

Preoperative Preparation of the Patient

Hip prep. Extends from toes to nippleline to at least 3 inches beyond midline back and front, including complete pubic area. Clean and trim toenails. Use brush on foot and nails. Hip fractures — all preps done in the operating room.

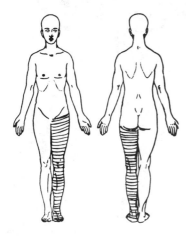

Knee and lower leg prep. Extends from entire leg, toes to groin. Clean and trim toenails. Use brush on foot and nails.

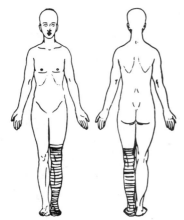

Ankle and foot prep. Extends from entire leg, toes to 3 inches above the knee. Clean and trim toenails. Use brush on foot and nails.

Table 6-1
Commonly Used Incisions

Incision	Location

Incision	Location
Collar (A)	Lower portion of the neck
Sternal split (B)	Midline over the sternum
Lateral thoracotomy (C)	Either enterolateral or postlateral aspects of the chest
Kocher's subcostal (D, E)	Oblique subcostal, right or left
Horizontal flank (F)	Midabdomen — right or left

Characteristics	Use
Letter	Key (Incision)
A	Collar
B	Sternal split
C	Lateral thoracotomy
D	Right subcostal
E	Left subcostal
F	Horizontal flank
G	Upper abdominal midline
H	Lower abdominal midline
I	Right upper paramedian
J	Right lower paramedian
K	Left upper paramedian
L	Left lower paramedian
M	McBurney's
N	Inguinal
O	Infraumbilical
P	Transverse upper abdominal
Q	Transverse suprapubic (Pfannenstiel)

Characteristics	Use
Provides adequate access to thyroid; generally heals well	Thyroid
Access overrides all other considerations	Cardiac procedures
Leaves quite a scar	
Generally heals well; incisions are necessarily long	Thoracic, cardiac procedures
Damage to an intercostal nerve can cause persistent pain in the scar	
Gives excellent exposure of upper abdominal contents; executed slowly and difficult to extend; very painful postoperatively; very unlikely to dehisce	Right side: gallbladder and biliary tract surgery Left side: surgery of the spleen
Allows access to the retroperitoneal space; is quickly	Lumbar sympathectomy Nephrectomy

(continued)

Table 6-1 (Continued)
Commonly Used Incisions

Incision	Location
Horizontal flank (F) (continued)	
Upper abdominal midline (G)	Upper abdomen— vertical
Lower abdominal midline (H)	Lower abdominal— vertical
Paramedian: Right upper and lower (I, J)	Upper or lower abdomen, a vertical incision to right of midline
Left upper and lower (K, L)	Upper or lower abdomen, a vertical incision to left of midline
McBurney's (M)	Over McBurney's point in right lower quadrant
Inguinal (N)	Inguinal region—right or left
Infraumbilical (O)	Below the umbilicus
Transverse upper abdominal (P)	Across the epigastric region
Transverse suprapubic (Pfannenstiel—Q)	Curved across and above the pubic arch

Characteristics	Use
executed, easily extended, and quickly closed	Ureterolithotomy
Provides a secure wound	Inferior vena cava ligation
Gives excellent exposure of upper abdominal contents; is quickly executed, easily extended, and quickly closed	Rapid entry into abdomen
	Gastrectomy
Not a strong incision, watch for signs and symptoms of dehiscence	
Gives excellent exposure of pelvic organs; is easily extended, and quickly closed, but not as strong as a transverse or paramedian lower abdominal incision	Hysterectomy
	Suprapubic prostatectomy
	Cystostomy
	Salpingectomy
	Presacral neurectomy
Gives excellent exposure to organs in a specific location; is slowly executed, easily extended. Provides a firm closure, unlikely to dehisce	Depends on location:
	Right upper paramedian: Biliary tract surgery
	Right lower paramedian: Appendectomy Small bowel resection Surgery on right adnexae
	Left upper paramedian: Surgery on the spleen Gastrectomy Vagectomy
	Left lower paramedian: Sigmoid colon resection Miles' resection Hysterectomy Surgery on left adnexae
Is quickly executed but difficult to extend, and gives poor exposure	Appendectomy
Gives a firm wound closure; unlikely to dehisce	
Does not enter abdomen	Repair of inguinal hernia
	Excision of hydrocele of spermatic cord
Is curvilinear	Only for umbilical hernia repair
Difficult to extend; hard to heal; painful postoperatively	Abdominal exploration
	Hiatal hernia repair
Difficult to extend; offers superior healing; has minimal tendency to disrupt; camouflaged in wrinkle line	Procedures on uterus, tubes, ovaries, and prostate

| **Surgical Instruments**

There are four basic categories of surgical instruments: sharps, clamps, graspers, and retractors. Each type has a specific purpose and is manufactured in a variety of sizes and shapes.

Sharps are used to incise and dissect tissue and bone. They include scalpels, scissors, bone cutters, rongeurs, chisels, osteotomes, saws, curettes, and dermatomes. Figure 6-2 pictures some of these instruments.

By controlling bleeding and maintaining homeostasis, clamps make surgery possible. They prevent excessive or fatal blood loss during dissection. The grasping end of a clamp has meshed serrations that prevent it from slipping off a blood vessel. Figure 6-3 illustrates a variety of clamps used in surgical procedures.

As their name implies, graspers grab and hold tissue or bone for dissection, retraction, or suturing. Graspers include tissue forceps, rib approximators, stone forceps, bone holders, sponge forceps, towel clips, needle holders, and other specialized instruments. Figure 6-4 pictures three types of grasping instruments.

Retractors are used to provide the best possible exposure of the operative site, while minimally traumatizing surrounding tissue. As Figure 6-5 shows, retractors can be self-retaining or handheld.

Lasers are being used more frequently in surgery, particularly in procedures where standard techniques for homeostasis or excision are ineffective, traumatic, or time-consuming. Despite certain disadvantages, such as their

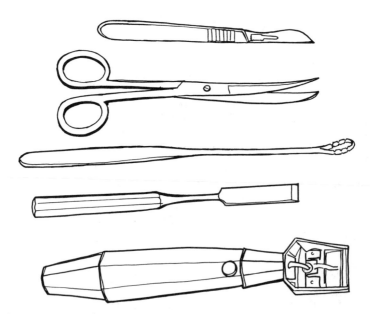

Figure 6-2. A variety of sharps

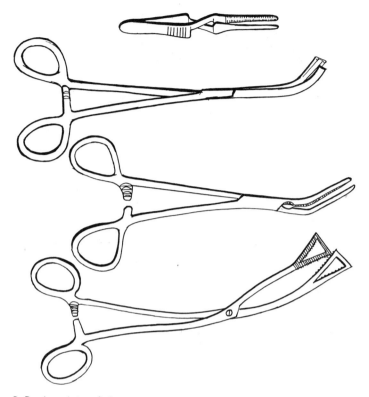

Figure 6-3. A variety of clamps

bulk, relative immobility, downtime, and expense, the use of lasers will likely increase. Surgical laser technology is rapidly advancing, while becoming less expensive. For example, multiple wavelengths are available with specific absorption by each tissue. Adjusting the energy applied varies the effect from massive destruction of a tumor to the ablation of a few cells.

Currently, argon, carbon dioxide, and neodymium (Nd) YAG (yttrium aluminium garnet) lasers produce the three wavelengths in general use. Each has a specific surgical effect. For example, the argon laser coagulates superficial vessels less than 1.5 mm diameter. Because water in the cells absorbs the carbon dioxide laser, it is very useful in removing neurological tumors. The Nd:YAG laser, which coagulates effectively and penetrates to a depth of 4 to 5 mm, is used to coagulate large vessels, vaporize tumors, and penetrate clots. Listed on page 154 are some applications of laser surgery.

| **Wound Closure**

The majority of surgical incisions are closed, either with or without drains or catheters in place. However, if grossly contaminated, a wound will be left

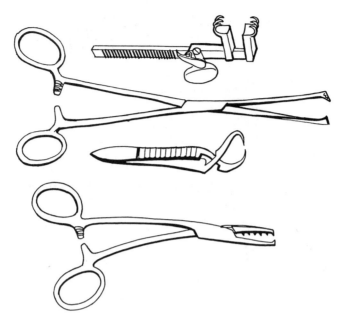

Figure 6-4. A variety of graspers

open. Since scar tissue is weaker and less elastic than normal tissue, the tissues are closely approximated to minimize the amount of scar tissue.

Sutures provide hemostasis, obliterate space, and give physical strength to a discontinuous surface. A variety of sutures, classified either as absorbable or nonabsorbable, are available for wound closure. Absorbable sutures are digested or hydrolyzed and assimilated by the tissues during the healing process. Conversely, nonabsorbable sutures are not absorbed by the tissues during the healing process. Nonabsorbable sutures, of which silk, cotton, nylon, polyester fiber, polypropylene, and stainless steel wire are examples, are most commonly used in suturing skin. A number of factors affect the choice of suture materials. These include the patient's history of wound healing, the operative site, the tissue involved, purpose of the suture, and the surgeon's experience.

Mechanical staplers are also used to ligate and divide, resect, anastomose, and close skin and fascia. Staplers are used in thoracic, abdominal, and gynecological surgery. Since tissue manipulation and handling are reduced, edema and inflammation are also reduced. The noncrushing shape of the "B" staples allows nutrition to pass to the tissue, thus decreasing the possibility of wound necrosis and retarded healing. In addition, since the staples are essentially nonreactive, the probability of tissue reaction or infection is also reduced.

Wound Drainage

Fluid collects in all surgical wounds during the healing process, but the amount varies, depending upon the procedure. Therefore, pressure dressings, drains, and closed wound suction are used to facilitate evacuation of the fluid. Drains, examples of which are pictured in Figure 6-6, are not brought out through the incision, but rather, through a separate stab wound because this decreases the infection rate.

Fluid drainage is either active or passive and depends upon several factors, including the type and extent of the surgical procedure, the amount and kind of drainage expected, and physician preference. In passive drainage, of which the Penrose drain is an example, drainage exists along the outside surface of the drain by capillary action. In active wound drainage, an external vacuum suction is connected to a drainage tube in a closed wound, thus creating suction in the wound. A sump drain is active drainage that uses a constant suction source and is open to the atmosphere. Conversely, a closed wound suction system is active drainage that uses a closed system. That is, it is not open to the atmosphere.

Closed wound suction, pictured in Figure 6-7, is used when a surgical

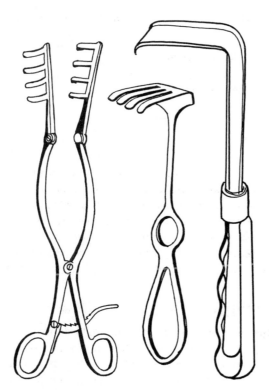

Figure 6-5. A variety of retractors

Applications of Laser Surgery

Otorhinolaryngology

    Treatment of tracheal stenosis

    Treatment of vocal cord papillomata

    Treatment of benign vocal cord tumors

    Treatment of leukoplakia of the oral mucosa

    Treatment of control multiple bleeding lesions of nasal passages

Plastic surgery

    Treatment of vascular skin lesions

    Removal of decorative tattoos

General surgery

    Control of GI bleeding

    Treatment of mucosal lesions of the GI tract

    Treatment of obstructive and bleeding carcinomas of esophagus, stomach, and rectum

Vascular surgery

    Excision of vascular tumor of the skin, tongue, head, and neck

Gynecological surgery

    Treatment of vulvar and cervical cancer

    Division of adhesions, opening of fimbriated end of the fallopian tube, and vaporization of endometriosis

procedure is expected to produce copious amounts of drainage, or when a "dry" wound is vital. Accumulations of large amounts of fluid become a bacterial medium. In addition, they impede wound healing by preventing the apposition of wound edges. They put pressure on surrounding organs and impede blood flow to the area. The result is necrosis of wound margins, the cutting of skin by sutures, postoperative infection, and an increase in postoperative pain. Therefore, closed wound suction is used in various neurologic, abdominal, orthopedic, urological, gynecological, and plastic procedures.

Dressings

Dressings applied at the end of a surgical procedure fulfill the following functions. They protect the incision from contamination and trauma; absorb drainage; support, splint, or immobilize the body part and the incision; facilitate hemostasis; minimize edema, and enhance the patient's physical and esthetic, or psychological, comfort.

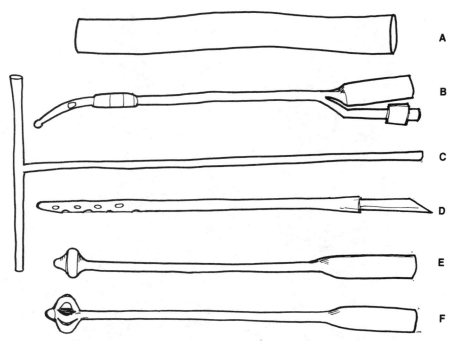

Figure 6-6. Types of drains. (A) Penrose drain. (B) Foley catheter. (C) "t" tube. (D) Saratoga sump drain. (E) Pezzar (mushroom) catheter. (F) Malecot (batwing) catheter.

Although the fibrin seals the incision within several hours after it is closed, a three-layer postoperative dressing is usually applied. The innermost layer, that next to the skin, is a nonadherent material. Therefore, when the dressing is removed, the healing process is not disrupted. The middle layer, usually gauze, collects blood products and debris, and the outer layer protects the wound.

The skin incision may be covered with a synthetic permeable membrane such as Op-Site. This thin, self-adhesive elastic film acts as a temporary second skin and provides a moist environment that is optimum for rapid and effective healing. Because the synthetic membrane is permeable to vapor and gases but not to liquids and bacteria, the wound is continuously bathed in serous exudate and healing is enhanced. Since the dressing can be easily removed without disrupting the newly formed epithelium, scar formation is minimized.

Transfer to the Postanesthesia Recovery Room

Once the patient's surgery is over, he is carefully moved from the operating room table to a stretcher or bed. This is a very critical time for the patient. Any

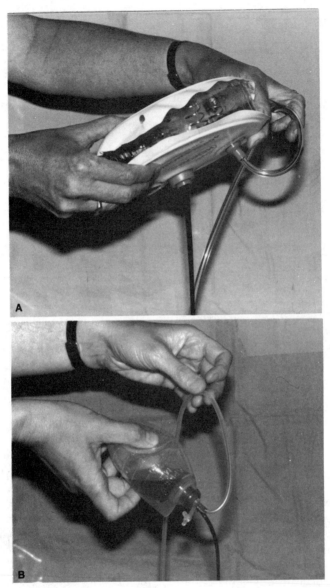

Figure 6-7. Two types of closed wound suction. (A) Hemovac drain. (B) Jackson
Pratt drain.

sudden or rough movement can cause his blood pressure to drop precipi-
tously, and he may even experience cardiac or respiratory arrest. The operating
room team is acutely aware of the patient's vulnerability and constantly alert
to potential complications.

Once the patient has been safely moved from the table, he is wheeled into the postanesthesia recovery room, accompanied by the circulating nurse and anesthesiologist. They explain the events of the patient's intraoperative experience and also convey relevant information gathered during the preoperative phase. Consequently, the postanesthesia recovery room nurse has a picture of the patient's perioperative experience to date, including the preoperative and intraoperative phases.

Evaluation

The patient remains free of injury and infection.

Summary

Many preparatory steps precede the surgeon's incision. Preparation for surgery begins in the preoperative phase with patient assessment and preparation and culminates in the intraoperative phase. By ensuring that the proper supplies and equipment are available and that all members of the surgery team follow surgical aseptic technique, the operating room nurse facilitates an uneventful intraoperative experience for the patient. Similarly, the skills and knowledge of the entire surgical team contribute to a complication-free recovery. Outcome criteria appropriate for a patient in the intraoperative phase are listed below.

Outcome Criteria for a Patient in the Intraoperative Phase

1. The patient is free of neuromuscular damage
2. The patient's skin is intact
3. The patient is free of injury as exhibited by correct needle, sponge, and instrument counts
4. The patient is hemodynamically stable
5. The patient's breathing pattern is symmetrical
6. The patient's peripheral tissues remain adequately perfused

From Kim MJ, McFarland GK, McLane AM (eds): Pocket Guide to Nursing Diagnoses. St. Louis, CV Mosby, 1984

References

1. Seropian R, Reynolds BM: Wound infections after preoperative depilatory versus razor preparation. Am J Surg 121: 251–254, March 1971

2.   Cruse PJE, Foord R: A five-year prospective study of 23,649 surgical wounds. Arch Surg 107: 206–210, 1973
3.   Balthazar EF, Colt JD, Nichols RL; Preoperative hair removal: A random prospective study of shaving versus clipping. South Med J 75(7): 799–801, 1982

Bibliography

Association of Operating room Nurses, Inc.: AORN Standards and Recommended Practices for Perioperative Nursing. Denver, The Association of Operating Room Nurses, 1983

Balthazar ER, Colt JD, Nichols RL: Preoperative hair removal: A random prospective study of shaving versus clipping. South Med J 75(7): 799–801, 1982

Besst JA, Wallace HL: Wound healing—Intraoperative factors. Nurs Clin North Am 14(4): 701–711, December 1979

Cruse PJE, Foord R: A five-year prospective study of 23,649 surgical wounds. Arch Surg 107: 206–210, 1973

Dixon JA: Surgical applications of lasers. AORN J 38(2): 223–230, August 1983

Garner JS: Guideline for Prevention of Surgical Wound Infections, 1985. Atlanta, U.S. Department of Health and Human Services, Public Health Service and Centers for Disease Control, 1985

Geelhoed GW, Sharpe K, Simon GL: A comparative study of surgical skin preparation methods. Surg Gynecol Obstet 157: 265–268, September 1983

Groah LK: Operating Room Nursing—the Perioperative Role. Reston, VA, Reston Publishing, 1983

Gruendemann BJ, Meeker MH: Alexander's Care of the Patient in Surgery, 7th ed. St. Louis, CV Mosby, 1983

Kneedler, JA, Dodge G: Perioperative Patient Care. Boston, Blackwell Scientific Publications, 1983

LeMaitre GD, Finnegan JA: The patient in Surgery: A Guide for Nurses, 4th ed. Philadelphia, WB Saunders, 1980

Mackety CJ: Perioperative Laser Nursing. Thorofare, NJ, SLACK Incorporated, 1984

McConnell EA: Clinical Considerations in the Use of Argyle Vac-U-Care Closed Wound Suction Systems. St. Louis, Argyle, 1983

Preoperative Depilation (editorial). The Lancet 1311, June 1983

Seropian R, Reynolds BM: Wound infections after preoperative depilatory versus razor preparation. Am J Surg 121: 251–254, March 1971

Westaby S: Wound care no. 5. Nurs Times 78: 17–20, January 20/26, 1982

Westaby S: Wound care no. 6. Nurs Times 78: 21–24, January 17/23, 1982

Yoder ME: Nursing diagnosis: Applications in perioperative practice. AORN J 40(2): 183–188, August 1984

Section 3
The Postoperative Phase

Eternal vigilance is the price of safety.

7 | The Postanesthesia Recovery Room

When you breathe you inspire, when you do not you expire

Many times the patient is in greater danger immediately *after* surgery than he is *during* surgery. His respiratory and circulatory processes are susceptible to changes, and lack of oxygen, as well as pain and sudden movement, can disrupt his physiologic equilibrium. He depends upon the postanesthesia recovery room nurse to meet his physiologic and emotional needs and to prevent the development of complications.

Admission to the Postanesthesia Recovery Room

Patient Assessment

The anesthesiologist and another member of the surgical team accompany the patient to the recovery room. They stay at the patient's bedside until the recovery room nurse assesses his respiratory and cardiovascular status.

Since the patient's well-being depends upon adequate ventilation, evaluation of airway patency is the single most important assessment the nurse makes when the patient is admitted to the recovery room. She auscultates the lungs, observes chest movement, and feels the flow of expired gases with her hand. Additionally, she evaluates the color of mucous membranes, level of consciousness, pulse rate and rhythm, and blood pressure. Oxygen should be given to all patients in the recovery room and is started as soon as possible.

When the recovery room nurse is satisfied that the patient's respiratory and cardiovascular status are adequate, the members of the surgical team describe the patient's intraoperative experience. The data they provide are listed on this and the opposite pages. Some of this information is found on the patient's anesthesia record (Figure 7-1) as well as on the operative record (Figure 7-2). The latter also contains the operating room nurses' record.

| **Nursing Diagnoses**

Once the postanesthesia recovery room nurse has assessed the patient and received a report from members of the surgical team, she identifies nursing

---

Data Provided Upon a Patient's Admission to the Postanesthesia Recovery Room

Patient's name, sex, age, and native language

Current medical diagnosis

Nature and length of the surgical procedure and responsible surgeon

Preoperative course:

    Vital signs

    Medications

    Potential or actual drug allergies

    Significant preoperative history

        Medical problems

        Medical history

        Communication handicaps

    Psychosocial

Intraoperative Course:

    Position in which patient was placed

    Vital signs

    Duration of tourniquet use

    Medications

        Preoperative medication
        Anesthetic

        Narcotic

        Narcotic Antagonist

        Muscle Relaxant

        Muscle relaxant reversal agent

        Antibiotic(s)

Other
Complications occurring during surgery
   Nature
   Treatment
Fluid therapy
   Estimated blood loss (EBL)
   Amount and kind of fluid administered
   Lines, site, patency ,and type of fluid being administered
      Peripheral
      Arterial
      Central Venous
      Swan-Ganz
   Urine output
Drains and catheters
   Type
   Number
Condition of wound
   Open
   Closed
   Packed
Condition of patient at end of procedure
   Vital Signs
   Presence of Prosthesis

diagnoses, derives goals, develops a plan to meet the goals, and implements and evaluates the plan. Nursing diagnoses applicable to the patient immediately after surgery are listed on page 166. Additionally, the nurse may incorporate plans initiated in the pre- and intraoperative phases so as to meet the patient's continuing needs. Although each diagnosis identified is associated with its own goal, the general goal of the immediate postanesthesia period is to ensure a safe and uneventful recovery.

| **Recovery Time**

Recovery from general anesthesia takes longer than induction for a number of reasons. During induction, the anesthetic is absorbed from the blood by tissues, particularly those that are highly vascular. During maintenance, anesthetic uptake occurs in muscle and fat. When administration of the agent is stopped, its blood level drops. Initially elimination is rapid because the alveolar walls are highly permeable to anesthetics. However fat, with its sparse

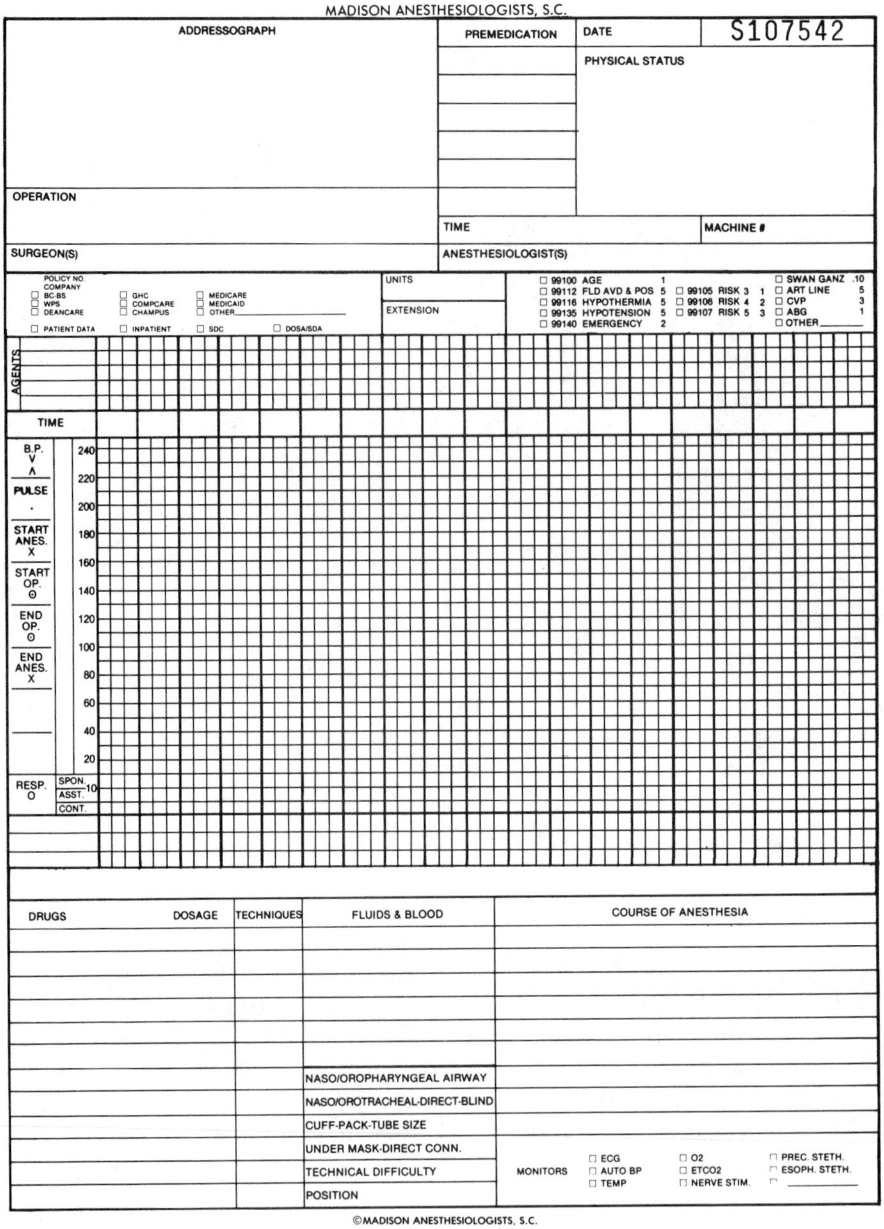

MADISON ANESTHESIOLOGISTS, S.C.

ADDRESSOGRAPH		PREMEDICATION	DATE	S107542
			PHYSICAL STATUS	

OPERATION

TIME		MACHINE #

SURGEON(S)

ANESTHESIOLOGIST(S)

POLICY NO.
COMPANY
☐ BC-BS
☐ WPS
☐ DEANCARE
☐ GHC
☐ COMPCARE
☐ CHAMPUS
☐ MEDICARE
☐ MEDICAID
☐ OTHER _____
☐ PATIENT DATA ☐ INPATIENT ☐ SDC ☐ DOSA/SDA

UNITS

EXTENSION

☐ 99100 AGE 1
☐ 99112 FLD AVD & POS 5
☐ 99116 HYPOTHERMIA 5
☐ 99135 HYPOTENSION 5
☐ 99140 EMERGENCY 2
☐ 99105 RISK 3 1
☐ 99106 RISK 4 2
☐ 99107 RISK 5 3
☐ SWAN GANZ .10
☐ ART LINE 5
☐ CVP 3
☐ ABG 1
☐ OTHER _____

AGENTS

TIME

B.P. ∨ ∧ 240, 220, 200, 180, 160, 140, 120, 100, 80, 60, 40, 20

PULSE .

START ANES. X

START OP. ⊙

END OP. ⊙

END ANES. X

RESP. ○   SPON. -10   ASST.   CONT.

DRUGS	DOSAGE	TECHNIQUES	FLUIDS & BLOOD	COURSE OF ANESTHESIA
		NASO/OROPHARYNGEAL AIRWAY		
		NASO/OROTRACHEAL-DIRECT-BLIND		
		CUFF-PACK-TUBE SIZE		
		UNDER MASK-DIRECT CONN.		
		TECHNICAL DIFFICULTY		MONITORS
		POSITION		

MONITORS
☐ ECG   ☐ O2   ☐ PREC. STETH.
☐ AUTO BP   ☐ ETCO2   ☐ ESOPH. STETH.
☐ TEMP   ☐ NERVE STIM.   ☐ _____

©MADISON ANESTHESIOLOGISTS, S.C.

Figure 7-1. Patient's anesthesia record.

OPERATIVE REGISTER

MADISON GENERAL HOSPITAL
MADISON, WISCONSIN

PREOPERATIVE
DIAGNOSIS:

POST-OPERATIVE
DIAGNOSIS:

| COMPLICATIONS: | DATE (17-22) | M | M | D | D | Y | Y |

OPERATION: | PROCEDURE (23-24) ROOM | | | | | 01-13-OR (1-13) 14-15-X-RAY (10-11) 99-OTHER

SURGEON: | SCHEDULE (25-28) TIME | HRS | MIN

RESIDENT: | ANESTHESIA (30-33) START TIME

ANESTHETIST: | PREPARATION: POSITION START TIME (35-38)

SCRUB PERSON 1 | OPERATION (40-43) START TIME

2 | OPERATION (45-48) STOP TIME

CIRCULATING PERSON 1 | PAR (50-53) START TIME

2 | PAR (55-58) STOP TIME

REMOVE TOP TWO COPIES BEFORE COMPLETING

SPONGE COUNT | PROC. (60-64) | SURG. (65-68) | ANEST. (69-72)

NEEDLE COUNT | RES. (73) 1. YES 2. NO | CLASS (75) | PT. TYPE (76) | SURG. (77) | AGE (78)

'EP SC

INSTRUMENT COUNT | ANES. (74) 1. GEN 2. LOC 3. NONE | 1 - CLASS I 2 - CLASS II 3 - CLASS III 4 - CLASS IV | 1. INPAT. 2. OUTPAT. 3. DAY CARE 5. DOSA | 1 SCHEDULED 2 UNSCHEDULED | 1 0-17 2 18-64 3 65-OVER

647-12 818211   10-84

183095

APPLIANCES AND PROSTHESIS _____

LOAD # _____ STERILIZER # _____ N/A _____

TIME	NURSES NOTES	TIME	MEDICATION	RT	SITE	SIGNATURE

PRIMARY NURSE _____   SURGEON _____
                        SIGNATURE   SIGNATURE

647-12 818211   **OPERATING ROOM NURSES RECORD**   10-84
                                                              PATIENT COPY

Figure 7-2. Operating room nurses' record. (Courtesy Madison General Hospital, Madison, WI)

Nursing Diagnoses Applicable in the Immediate Postanesthetic Phase

Potential for ineffective airway clearance related to decreased level of consciousness

Potential for impaired gas exchange related to hypoventilation

Potential for decreased cardiac output related to rapid position change

Potential for fluid volume deficit related to: Decreased fluid intake; abnormal fluid loss

Potential for fluid volume excess related to fluids received in surgery

Potential for injury related to sensory deficits

Alteration in comfort related to acute pain

From Kim MJ, McFarland GK, McLane AM (eds): Pocket Guide to Nursing Diagnoses. St. Louis, CV Mosby, 1984

---

blood supply, gives up the anesthetic agent more slowly. Other factors affecting a patient's recovery time include the preoperative medications administered and the anesthetic agent, including length of administration, dosage in relation to the patient's body size, and the body's response to the agent.

Return of Reflexes

When a patient recovers from a general anesthetic, his reflexes return in the reverse order in which they disappeared. The usual sequence of return is:

> Unconsciousness
> Response to stimuli
> Drowsiness
> Awake but not oriented
> Alert and oriented.

The patient first responds with motor or reflex activity to a stimulus such as having his eyelid touched. As more of the anesthetic dissipates, the patient becomes oriented, first to person, and then to place and time.

When the patient awakens, voices may seem quite loud. His thoughts are fuzzy and unclear and his vision is often blurred. Next, he notices that his arms and legs feel heavy. He wonders where he is and feels things in his mouth. Although still likely to be drowsy and disoriented to place and time, he may realize that he hurts, depending upon the medications he received intraoperatively.

The nurse reorients the patient frequently and when doing so calls him by his preferred name. Otherwise, the patient may not realize that the nurse is speaking to him.

The nurse speaks to the patient in a normal voice, while standing close to his head. When speaking to the patient she touches him so that he knows that she is there to care for him. However, if the patient received ketamine intraoperatively, the nurse provides him with a quiet recovery area since hallucinations and excitement can occur on emergence. She avoids touching him.

Since hearing is the first sense to return, the nurse not only tells the patient when she is going to do something to him, but also avoids careless conversation while with and around him. Because the patient is semiconscious he may misinterpret comments and become frightened.

Usually within an hour after arriving in the recovery room the patient becomes oriented to person, place, and time. He may fall asleep when not stimulated, but readily responds when spoken to or touched.

The average recovery room stay is less than 2 hours, due primarily to the short-acting anesthetics used. During the patient's stay, the recovery room nurse reassesses him every 10 to 15 minutes initially, and then as his condition warrants. She documents her observations and actions on a postanesthesia record such as illustrated in Figure 7-3. Throughout the patient's stay, the nurse meets his physiologic and emotional needs via observations and appropriate interventions. (See the listing elsewhere on this page.)

Observations and Interventions in the Postanesthesia Recovery Room

1. Check airway; feel for the amount of air exchange. If oxygen is to be administered, start it at flow rate ordered. Note rate, depth, and quality of respirations.

2. Note presence or absence of protective throat reflexes.

3. Obtain pulse and blood pressure readings. Note rate and quality of pulse. Compare all vital sign readings with patient's preoperative and intraoperative values.

4. Determine patient's level of consciousness.

5. Observe the patient's skin color; check the mucous membrane inside the lower lip and also his nail beds.

6. Note any I.V. infusions: type and amount of fluid infusing, rate of infusion, position of needle, and location of site.

7. Observe the presence and condition of any drains and tubes. Be sure they are not kinked or occluded and are properly attached to suction or a drainage bag.

8. Assess any dressings. If they are soiled, note the color, type, odor, and amount of the drainage.

9. Note the amount and type of any irrigant infusing.

10. Observe factors specific to the surgery.

11. Take the patient's temperature.

12. Encourage patient to take deep breaths and move his legs, unless contraindicated, three to four times every 15 minutes.

13. Reassure the patient that surgery is over and that he is in the recovery room.

14. Review doctor's orders: administer medications, as ordered.

15. Note observations and interventions on the postanesthesia record.

| Respiratory and Cardiovascular Function

Respiration is the exchange of oxygen and carbon dioxide between the atmosphere and cells of the body. The respiratory process includes ventilation, diffusion, and transportation. That is, the patient inhales and exhales; oxygen diffuses from the pulmonary alveoli to the blood and carbon dioxide, from the blood to the alveoli; and oxygen is transported to and carbon dioxide from the body cells.

Adequate tissue oxygenation depends upon adequate respiratory function, as well as upon normal cardiovascular function. These two functions are interdependent.

The main function of the cardiovascular system is transport. Normal cardiovascular function is essential to transport oxygen from the lungs to the cells and carbon dioxide from the cells to the lungs. This gas transport system involves the heart, the arteries, capillaries, veins, and the blood and its components. The heart acts as a pump, the arteries, capillaries, and veins as conducting pathways, and the blood as the transport medium. An alteration in any of these factors can disrupt cardiovascular function and cardiac output.

Inadequate Respiratory Function

The two major causes of inadequate respiratory function in the immediate postoperative period and the two most common causes of postoperative hypoxemia are airway obstruction and hypoventilation. Hypercarbia often accompanies hypoxemia and is usually secondary to inadequate ventilation.

The major causes of airway obstruction are the tongue and secretions. Depression of the pharyngeal reflexes allows the tongue to drop into the throat and obstruct the airway. Similarly, secretions obstruct the airway by collecting in the pharynx, trachea, or bronchial tree. Other causes of airway obstruction include laryngeal spasm, edema, blood, mucus plugs, and vomitus.

Vomiting is not uncommon in patients recovering from general anesthesia and is dangerous. Passive vomiting is particularly dangerous because it occurs with little noticeable gagging. Vomitus, if aspirated, can cause severe

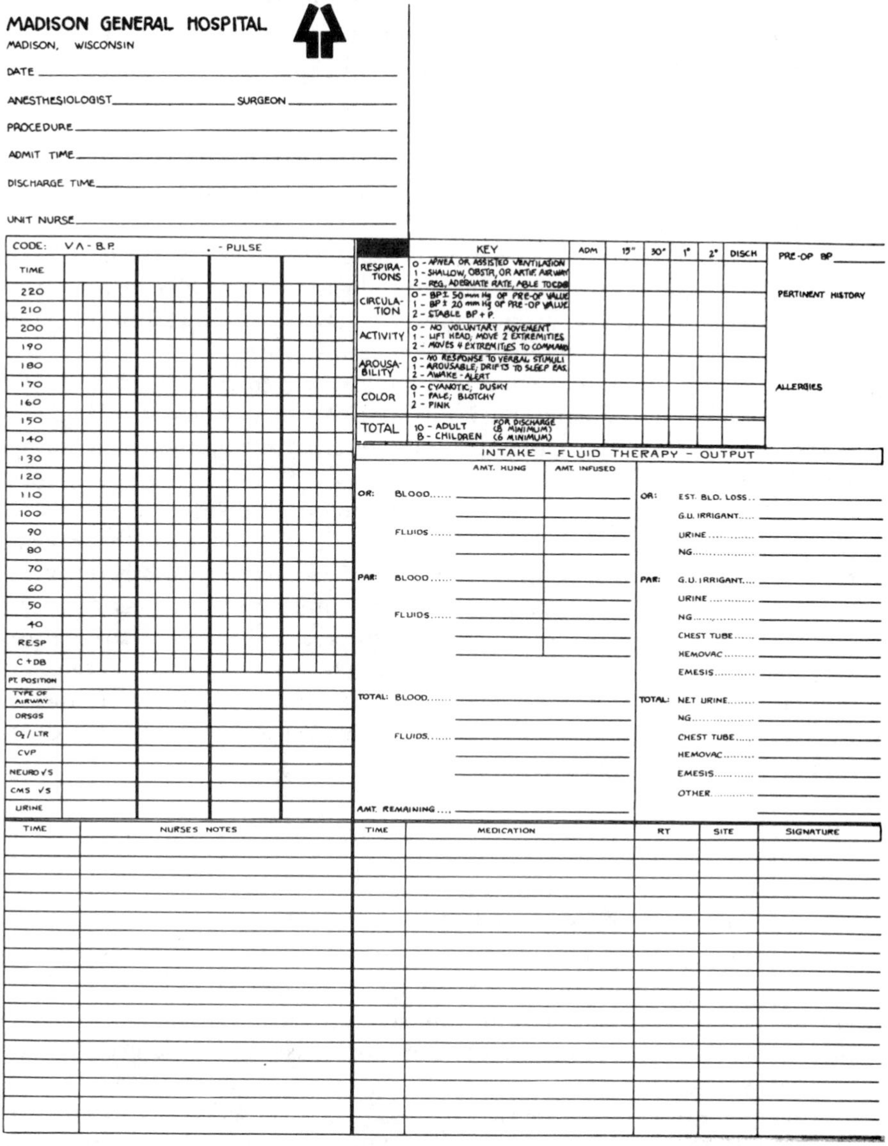

Figure 7-3. Patient's postanesthesia record. (Courtesy Madison General Hospital, Madison, WI)

pulmonary complications such as pneumonitis, destruction of lung tissue, pulmonary edema, and respiratory failure. Aspiration is a major cause of death associated with anesthesia (See Chapter 8).

Restlessness and a rapid, thready pulse are early signs of respiratory distress. Cyanosis, on the other hand, is not only a late sign, but also an unreliable sign because the patient's circulatory status, his temperature, and room light affect it. Other signs and symptoms of respiratory distress include

Rapid, shallow respirations

Reduced tidal volume

Attempting to sit upright

Flaring nares

Excessive use of the accessory breathing muscles in the abdomen, neck and chest

Retraction of the intercostal spaces and tissues of the neck.

Noisy respirations such as snoring and gasping also indicate respiratory distress but do not always accompany obstructed breathing. However, noisy respirations *always* demand immediate investigation.

In hypoventilation a reduced amount of air enters the pulmonary alveoli. A common problem in the immediate postanesthetic period, hypoventilation may occur in any patient who has received an anesthetic, including a spinal anesthetic.

Causes of postoperative hypoventilation can be divided into two broad categories, those related to events of the intraoperative phase and those related to the patient's physical condition. The residual effects of anesthetic agents, narcotics, tranquilizers, sedatives, and neuromuscular relaxants can cause respiratory depression in the immediate postoperative period, as can decreased stimulation. Factors inherent in the patient's physical condition that can cause respiratory depression include obesity, advanced age, chronic lung disease, liver disease, and cardiovascular disease. Other causes include gastric dilatation and a constricting surgical dressing.

Disrupted Cardiovascular Function

Dysrhythmias and hypotension commonly occur in the immediate postoperative period. Although a variety of factors, including hypokalemia, pain, hypovolemia, gastric distention, and acidosis, can cause cardiac dysrhythmias, hypoxemia and hypercarbia are the common causes of premature beats and sinus tachycardia.

Hypotension in the immediate postoperative period can result from anesthetic agents, hypoxemia, cardiac dysrhythmias, narcotics, and rapid changes in body position. However, hypovolemia is the most common cause.

During surgery a balance between vasodilation and vasoconstriction keeps the patient's blood pressure within normal limits. Anesthetic agents such as halothane cause peripheral vasodilation that results in mild hypotension, while surgery produces sympathetic vasoconstriction. After surgery the patient's blood pressure normally drops slightly. This drop is usually well tolerated by healthy patients and is not treated.

Maintaining Respiratory and Cardiovascular Function

Adequate respiratory and cardiovascular function depend upon a patent airway, adequate ventilation, an efficient and effective heart, and adequate fluid volume. The postanesthesia recovery room nurse uses various interventions to ensure adequate respiratory and cardiovascular function. These include managing artificial airways, administering oxygen, properly positioning the patient, encouraging respiratory exercises, removing secretions, minimizing hypothermia, and administering reversal agents and intravenous fluids.

Artificial Airways

Tracheal and pharyngeal airways, as pictured in Figure 7-4, help maintain a patent airway. Neither is removed until the reflexes for controlling coughing and swallowing have returned.

A tracheal airway connects the patient's trachea to anesthetic gases during surgery and later to room air or oxygen via tubing. It prevents the tongue and foreign bodies from obstructing the patient's airway and may also prevent laryngeal spasm from occluding it.

A tracheal airway, such as an endotracheal tube, is not removed until the patient is awake and able to maintain his own airway. In addition, if he received a neuromuscular blocking agent during surgery, he must regain muscular control before being extubated. That is, he must be able to raise his head from a supine position (unless contraindicated by the surgical procedure) and squeeze and release the nurse's hand on command. Other criteria for successful extubation are

1. Regular respiratory pattern
2. Respiratory rate between 10 and 35
3. Tidal volume >5 ml per kilogram
4. Vital capacity >15 ml per kilogram
5. Arterial carbon dioxide tension <45 mm Hg
6. Arterial oxygen tension >60 mm Hg on room air[1]

Pharyngeal airways, either oropharyngeal or nasal pharyngeal, prevent the tongue from relaxing into the throat. However, an oropharyngeal airway is by no means foolproof. Its position may change if the patient's jaw drops or if he attempts to swallow. An oropharyngeal airway is removed when the patient begins to swallow or if it makes him gag or vomit. Patients tolerate nasal pharyngeal airways considerably longer than oropharyngeal and seldom gag even when they are moderately alert.

Oxygen Therapy

Oxygen is always given to treat hypoxemia, a common cause of cardiac dysrhythmias such as premature beats and sinus tachycardia. Practically all pa-

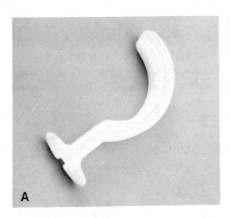

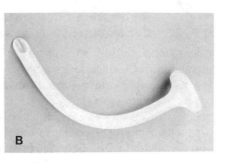

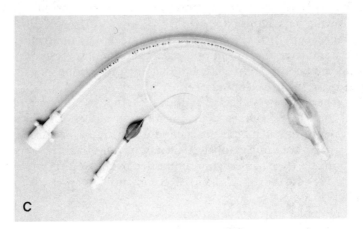

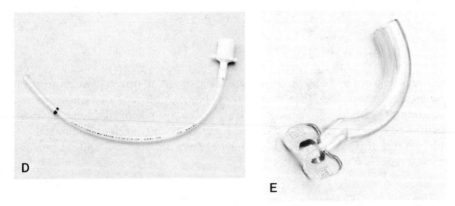

Figure 7-4. Artificial airways. (A) Berman oral airway. (B) Nasopharyngeal airway.
(C) Low pressure cuffed tracheal tube—oral/nasal. (D) Uncuffed
tracheal tube—oral/nasal. (E) Guedal oral airway. (Courtesy Portex,
Inc., Wilmington, MA)

tients receive high humidity oxygen immediately postoperatively because most hypoventilate when emerging from anesthesia.

The amount of oxygen administered depends upon the patient, the anesthesiologist, and institutional policy, but usually is between 40% and 60% with a flow rate between 6 L and 10 L. The percentage for patients with chronic obstructive pulmonary disease is lower, because for them the respiratory stimulus is a decrease in blood oxygen, not an elevation in carbon dioxide levels. The administration of a high concentration of oxygen obliterates their respiratory drive.

Patients usually receive oxygen until they are conscious and able to take deep breaths. Arterial blood gas determinations indicate when prolonged oxygen therapy is necessary. Regardless of its duration, oxygen therapy benefits the patient only when it reaches the lungs. Therefore, the airway must be patent.

Despite adequate ventilation and oxygenation, a patient may develop a cardiac dysrhythmia. The nurse determines how the patient is tolerating it and if he has a history of dysrhythmias. If the dysrhythmia existed preoperatively and has not changed, treatment will probably not be necessary. If the patient has no history of dysrhythmias, the nurse notifies the physician. Drugs such as intravenous lidocaine or procainamide may be administered, and atropine may be used to treat the sinus bradycardia caused by neostigmine and edrophonium.

Positioning

Properly positioning the patient's head, as well as the patient himself, can relieve pharyngeal obstruction. For example, backward tilt of the head and anterior displacement of the mandible can alleviate airway obstruction.

The ideal patient position ensures a patent airway and allows the patient to breathe normally, expanding all portions of the lungs. The position also facilitates the drainage of mucus, vomitus, and blood, and prevents aspiration.

The ideal position depends upon the surgery performed, the patient's size and condition, and the anesthesia used. For example, despite its disadvantages, the sitting position is recommended for patients having had a neck or chest procedure, esophagoscopy, thyroidectomy, laryngectomy, lung resection, bronchoscopy, or a radical neck dissection. Similarly, elevating the head of the bed, unless contraindicated by surgery, relieves pressure on the diaphragm of an obese patient.

For the majority of patients the lateral decubitus or semiprone position, with the head tilted back and the jaw supported forward, is best until such protective reflexes as coughing have returned. The lateral decubitus position helps prevent a sagging tongue from obstructing the airway and promotes drainage of secretions out of the mouth. Chest expansion, which is somewhat decreased in the lateral decubitus position, can be enhanced by turning the patient frequently and elevating and positioning the flexed upper arm on a pillow. Respiratory exchange in an awake patient with intact reflexes is improved in a head elevated/semisitting position, unless contraindicated by surgery.

Respiratory Exercises

Encouraging the patient to take three or four deep breaths to total lung capacity every 10 to 15 minutes and to hold each breath for at least 3 seconds has several advantages (See Chapter 3). It helps hyperinflate the alveoli, thus reversing the atelectasis that results from anesthesia inhalation and lying in one position during surgery. It enhances gaseous exchange and facilitates the elimination of anesthetic gases. And because voluntary deep breaths are an inspiratory maneuver, they are not painful.

Inspiratory maneuvers, such as deep breathing, yawning, and sighing, are more effective in preventing postoperative atelectasis than are expiratory maneuvers such as coughing. Inspiratory maneuvers inflate the alveoli and maintain a normal functional residual capacity.

Expiratory maneuvers, such as coughing, increase the pleural pressure above that of the airway. The alveoli deflate and the lung volume decreases. Coughing is indicated only when the patient has secretions and is contraindicated following certain procedures such as cataract removal, craniotomy, ear surgery, and repair of a large abdominal hernia.

If the patient cannot cough effectively, the nurse suctions him. Frequently, only phayrngeal suctioning is needed. However, if intratracheal suctioning is needed, sterile technique must be used, and the nurse hyperventilates the patient with 100% oxygen before and after each insertion of the catheter.

Voluntary deep breathing not only improves lung ventilation and helps ensure adequate respiratory function, but also improves cardiovascular status. By enhancing venous return to the heart, voluntary deep breathing helps empty the deep veins of the legs and minimizes peripheral pooling of blood.

Minimizing Hypothermia

Hypothermia and shivering are common in postoperative patients. Factors predisposing to hypothermia include advanced age, very young age, certain anesthetics, blood loss, the infusion of cold fluids, prolonged operating time, and saturated drapes. Surgery stresses the body's ability to maintain a normal temperature. The integrity of the skin is disturbed and both the interior and exterior of the body are exposed to unnatural and sometimes hostile environments, including cool operating room temperatures. In addition, anesthetics depress the thermoregulatory centers, and most anesthetic techniques cause vasodilation that increases heat loss. Although hypothermia itself may depress body activity and decrease oxygen demand, uncontrolled hypothermia can be fatal.

Severe shivering can greatly increase oxygen consumption. The rebound of shivering during recovery can increase oxygen consumption by 400%. Gross uncontrolled shivering can result in hypoxemia, hypercarbia, acidosis, and even cardiac arrest if muscle activity and hypoxemia persist.

Immediately postoperatively the nurse initiates measures for rewarming the patient. She removes wet, cold, linen from beneath the patient and covers him with blankets from an electric blanket storage warmer. In addition, she monitors the patient's temperature and unless contraindicated, administers oxygen until he stops shivering.

Keeping the patient warm not only makes him more comfortable, but also enhances his circulation. This is important because poor circulation inhibits transport, which ultimately results in poor excretion of the anesthetic.

Reversal Agents

Hypoventilation and respiratory depression in the immediate postoperative period may be drug-induced. Residual effects of opiate narcotics and neuromuscular blocking agents cause postoperative hypoventilation.

If a narcotic is responsible for respiratory depression, naloxone will be administered. Naloxone is the only narcotic antagonist that does not produce respiratory depression. That is, when administered to a patient whose respiratory depression is caused by barbiturates or other nonopoid drugs, naloxone simply fails to act. However, naloxone is not benign. The duration of naloxone's action ranges from 30 to 60 minutes, while that of narcotics is much longer, up to 4 or 5 hours. Therefore, respiratory depression may return as the effects of naloxone diminish.

Naloxone not only reverses the depressant effects narcotics, but also terminates their analgesic effects. Therefore, the patient may experience intense postoperative pain, accompanied by tachycardia, hypertension, and increased vascular resistance. Several cases of acute pulmonary edema, in otherwise healthy patients, have been reported following the use of naloxone.

Treatment of respiratory depression resulting from neuromuscular blocking agents depends upon whether a nondepolarizing or depolarizing agent was used. As Table 5-6 indicates, an anticholinesterase such as edrophonium or neostigmine is effective against nondepolarizing neuromuscular blocking agents such as d-tubocurarine and pancuronium.

A variety of factors prolong the effects of nondepolarizing neuromuscular blocking agents. These include diseases such as oat cell carcinoma, renal insufficiency, and cirrhosis; and electrolyte and acid-base imbalances such as hypokalemia, hypocalcemia, and respiratory acidosis. Additionally, the administration of quinidine, lidocaine, propranolol, and aminoglycosides during surgery and in the immediate postoperative period have caused muscular weakness. Manual or mechanical ventilation is used until normal function is restored.

If a depolorizing neuromuscular blocking agent such as succinylcholine is causing respiratory depression, continued mechanical ventilatory support is essential until its effects dissipate. An anticholinesterase should *never* be used to reverse succinylcholine because the enzyme can prolong the effect of the blocking agent. Patients with liver disease, who may have abnormally low levels of the enzyme pseudocholinesterase, are often more susceptible to respiratory depression from depolarizing agents than patients with normal levels of the enzyme.

Fluid Administration

Most patients receive intravenous fluids immediately postoperatively to maintain their fluid and electrolyte balance and to prevent hypovolemia and hypotension. The amount and kind of fluid administered depends upon the individual patient's need. Factors affecting this need include the patient's preoperative status, the surgery performed, the patient's intraoperative experience, and his response to stressors.

Third spacing, an especially important consideration in abdominal and other major surgery, represents a redistribution of isotonic fluid from functional to nonfunctional body compartments. Usually this is a transfer of extracellular fluid to an acute sequestered edema space. This "third space" is functionally part of interstitial fluid space, but is nonfunctional in that it is physiologically useless. An increase in body weight reflects this trapped fluid. Since the body cannot use this fluid, the patient can become relatively hypovolemic. Therefore, large volumes of fluid are given intraoperatively.

Third space fluid is usually mobilized 1 to 3 days after a trauma. The fluid returns to the extracellular fluid and is lost from the body as urine.

The nurse notes not only the kind and amount of fluid the patient receives in the postanesthesia recovery room, but also the kind and amount administered intraoperatively. She also monitors all output, including urine and drainage from tubes and dressings. Normal urinary output accurately predicts adequate perfusion and patient recovery. All tubes must be patent, kink-free, and properly functioning, and suction equipment must be operating appropriately. The nurse notes the color, consistency, odor, and amount of drainage from any tube. In addition, she notes the condition of all dressings. Are they dry or soiled? If soiled, what is the color, type, odor, and amount of the drainage?

Electrolytes are not routinely monitored in the immediate postoperative period unless major disturbances are suspected due to disease or intervention. For example, electrolyte determinations are essential immediately postoperatively if a major physiological fluid loss has occurred; if fluid administration has been mismanaged; or if a significant amount of liquid has been deliberately or accidentally administered.

Although glucose is not an electrolyte, serum glucose levels are frequently obtained in the immediate postoperative period of diabetics. The value determines the amount of insulin, or in some cases glucose, to be given.

Physical Safety and Physical and Emotional Comfort

The patient in the immediate postoperative period depends upon the nurse for his physical safety and physical and emotional well-being. Many events in the immediate postoperative period can cause the patient physical harm and physical and emotional discomfort. The patient is at risk for falls, and some patients are at risk for delirium. Pain and hypothermia can cause physical discomfort, while fear, anxiety, and confusion can cause emotional distress.

Some patients experience a near-delirium upon emerging from anesthesia. Wild thrashing and shouting can indicate emergence delirium. Although hypoxemia can trigger delirium, predisposing factors include the patient's age, his physical status, the type of surgery performed, pain, and certain drugs. Young, healthy, active, muscular patients, who have had surgery that they anticipated would be painful or mutilating, experience delirium reactions more often than older or debilitated patients. Severe pain or an adverse reaction to scopolamine or ketamine can also trigger delirium reactions.

Pain may be the patient's most serious postoperative problem and is whatever he says it is. By the time the patient arrives in the postanesthesia recovery room he may be experiencing pain, depending upon the surgery and the amount and kind of anesthetic administered. The amount of pain that he verbalizes may differ from that which he experiences. Factors affecting the patient's expression of pain include his psychological makeup, the relationship he has with his family, the size and location of the incision, the amount of organ manipulation involved, and the meaning of the procedure to him.

Pain not only causes the patient physical and emotional discomfort, but also can cause hypertension. Hypertension is a threat particularly to patients with cardiovascular disease. Other causes of hypertension include carbon dioxide retention and bladder distention.

Maintaining Physical Safety

Safety Measures

Side rails on the stretcher or bed must be raised and the knee straps loosely secured. In order to prevent nerve damage from pressure and joint and muscle strain from lying in one position, the patient's body is properly aligned. The nurse pads the metal side rails if they touch the patient and adds an extender to the stretcher if the patient is so tall that his feet hang over the edge. The extender prevents nerve damage.

The nurse turns the patient frequently, unless contraindicated. She pays particular attention to the unconscious patient and to the those recovering from spinal or epidural anesthesia. These patients have loss of sensation and are oblivious to discomfort.

Treatment of delirium generally requires patience and time. However, since restlessness is a well-known manifestation of hypoxemia, it is first excluded as a cause. Sedatives are usually ineffective because it is the combination of sedatives and postoperative pain that precipitate this agitation.

Maintaining Physical
and Emotional Comfort

A variety of nursing interventions ensure physical and emotional comfort. They include keeping the patient warm, administering pain medication, decreasing his anxiety, and protecting his dignity and privacy.

Pain Medication

Pain medication is given in the immediate postanesthesia period, but only after the nurse has carefully assessed the patient, reviewed the type of anesthetic used, and determined whether a reversing agent was administered at the end of the procedure. Since the effects of the anesthetic may not have completely worn off, the dose of the pain medication is usually reduced to one third to one quarter of the usual dose.

Narcotic analgesics are usually given intravenously. This route expedites pain relief and minimizes respiratory depression by giving the nurse more control over the medication (See Chapter 8 for more information about pain relief techniques).

In addition to relieving the patient's pain, the nurse also enhances his comfort by making sure that he is warm. She also removes excess tape and the electrodes, and provides mouth care.

Decreasing Anxiety

A nurse who is caring, reassuring, and calm can decrease the patient's anxiety and increase his emotional comfort. As soon as the patient arrives in the postanesthesia recovery room the nurse tells him that his surgery is over and that he is in the recovery room. She also tells him the time, a question patients frequently ask. Throughout the patient's stay, the nurse frequently reorients and reassures the patient.

Protecting Dignity and Privacy

The nurse protects the patient's dignity and privacy and includes his family in his care. She treats the patient respectfully and does not expose him unnecessarily. Soon after the patient arrives in the recovery room, the nurse telephones the patient's family to tell them that he has arrived.

Discharge from the Postanesthesia Recovery Room

A patient is discharged from the postanesthesia recovery room when it is deemed safe to do so. However, determining when a patient can be safely discharged depends upon the unit to which he is being transferred. The physical condition of a patient being transferred to an intensive care unit usually differs significantly from that of a patient being transferred to a general hospital unit; both differ from the condition of a patient being discharged to a one-day surgery unit. In all instances, however, patient safety is the major consideration.

Usually a scoring system, an example of which is included in Figure 7-3, is used to quantify the patient's physical status postoperatively. Unless limited by preoperative conditions, the patient should score high. Acutely ill patients and those not meeting the criteria listed on the opposite page are usually transferred to an intensive care unit.

Regardless of the unit to which the patient is to be discharged, the nurse who cares for him in the recovery room provides the patient's primary or unit nurse with a complete report of his immediate postanesthesia experience. Ideally, the recovery room nurse accompanies the patient during transfer. When this is not possible, she telephones the nurse to report significant information and to alert her to specific equipment ordered for the patient.

Outcome Criteria for a Person Discharged from the Postanesthesia Recovery Room to a Nonintensive care Unit

1. The patient must be able to protect his own airway.
2. The patient must be able to move in bed enough to turn his head to expel vomitus.
3. Respirations should be quiet and unlabored.
4. The patient must be able to clear any secretions.
5. The patient must be hemodynamically stable.
6. The patient's underlying medical diseases have been evaluated.
7. The patient must be able to summon help when needed.
8. The patient must be reasonably comfortable, but not overly sedated.
9. The surgical procedure must be reviewed before discharge.
10. Postsurgical complications have been evaluated and are under control.
11. Motor function and proprioception have returned for the patient who has undergone a regional anesthesia.

Evaluation

The patient recovers from the anesthesia without any complications.

Summary

Each patient is unique. Despite the fact that all patients in the immediate postanesthesia period share certain nursing diagnoses, goals, and interventions, routine postoperative patients simply do not exist.

The nurse reassesses each postoperative patient continuously throughout his recovery room stay. Her reassessments enable her to manage his care knowledgeably. Although "routine" orders are common in the postanesthesia recovery room, the nurse sees the patient as the unique person that he is and confidently intervenes to meet his physiologic and emotional needs.

References

1. Orkin LR, Shapiro G: Admission and assessment and general monitoring. Int Anesthesiol Clin 21(1):7 Spring 1983

Bibliography

Andrews DR, Taylor C: Documenting post-anesthesia recovery. Am J Nurs 85(3): 290–291, 1985

Borchardt AC, Fraulini KE: Hypothermia in the postanesthetic patient. AORN 36(4): 648–669, October 1982

Carey KW: Caring for Surgical Patients. Springhouse, PA, Intermed Communications, 1982

Cullen DJ: Recovery room care of the surgical patient. Int Anesthesiol Clin 18(3): 39–52, Fall 1980

Fraulini KE, Murphy P: R.E.A.C.T. A new system for measuring postanesthesia recovery. Nurs 84 14(4): 101–102.

Fraulini KE, Gorski DW: Don't let perioperative medications put you in a spin. Nurs 83 13(12): 26–30, 1983

Hartwell PW: Discharge criteria. Int Anesthesiol Clin 21(1): 107–14, Spring 1983

Hatridge L: Holding room in the O.R. a must. Point of View 21(3): 15, 1984

Hudelson, E: A 'just in case' guide to postanesthetic recovery for the non-recovery-room nurse. RN 45(3): 51–53, 1982

Julien R: Understanding Anesthesia. Menlo Park, CA, Addison-Wesley, 1984

Kim MJ, McFarland GK, McLane AM (eds): Pocket Guide to Nursing Diagnoses. St. Louis, CV Mosby, 1984

Kneedler JA, Dodge GE: Perioperative Patient Care. Boston, Blackwell Scientific Publications, 1983

LeMaitre GD, Finnegan JA: The Patient in Surgery: A Guide for Nurses, 4th ed. Philadelphia, WB Saunders, 1980

Lewis KP, Cressy I: Nursing care for postanesthesia shivering. AORN J 30(2): 357–362, August 1979

Long BC, Gowin CJ, Bushong ME: Surgical intervention. In Phipps WJ, Long BC, Woods NF (eds): Medical—Surgical Nursing, 2nd ed. St. Louis, CV Mosby, 1983

McConnell EA: After surgery. Nurs 83 13(2): 74–84, 1983

Orkin LR, Shapiro G: Admission assessment and general monitoring. Int Anesthesiol Clin 21(1): 3–12, Spring 1983

Ozuna JM, Foster C: Hypothermia and the surgical patient. Am J Nurs 79(4): 646–648, 1979

Pellegrini CA: Postoperative care. In Way LW (ed): Current Surgical Diagnosis and Treatment, 6th ed. Los Altos, CA, Lange Medical Publications, 1983

Seaman DJ: Shortcuts to a more complete postanesthesia room transfer. Nurs 83 13(9): 47–49, 1983

Sigg LV, Fallucca LL: Recognizing hypoventilation in the recovery room. AORN J 38(2): 270–285, August 1983

Sweeney SS: OR observations: Key to postop pain. AORN J 32(3): 391–400, September 1980

8 | Postoperative Complications and Their Prevention

> The objectives of the monitoring and the interpretation of the data remain more important than the equipment or hardware, and thus equal attention must be paid to electrical connections and synaptic functions.
>
> —Orkin and Shapiro

The patient's postoperative experience continues as he is transferred from the postanesthesia recovery room to his unit. The nurse greets him, receives reports from the recovery room nurse about his intra- and immediate postoperative experiences, and assesses him. These data provide the nurse with an inclusive and current view of the patient's perioperative experience. They enable her to identify postoperative complications for which he is at risk and to continue to plan with him for discharge.

Nursing Diagnoses

The many nursing diagnoses that are applicable to postoperative patients are identified from a combination of pre-, intra-, and immediate postoperative assessment data. From these data the nurse establishes goals, and develops, implements, and evaluates a plan of care appropriate to the individual patient. The most common nursing diagnoses applicable to patients in the postoperative phase are listed on page 182.

**Nursing Diagnoses Applicable to
Patients in the Postoperative Phase**

Potential for ineffective airway clearance related to ineffective cough reflex, postoperative pain, positioning

Potential for alteration in bowel elimination: Constipation related to narcotics, altered activity, changes in dietary patterns

Ineffective breathing pattern related to postoperative pain, incisional site

Alteration in comfort: Pain related to surgical incision, inadequate postoperative pain management

Alteration in fluid volume: Excess related to intravenous infusion rate

Potential alteration in fluid volume: Deficit related to loss of gastrointestinal secretions and wound drainage

Potential for impaired gas exchange related to retained secretions, hypoventilation due to incisional pain

Potential for injury related to nosocomial infection

Disturbance in self-concept related to alteration in body image

Potential alteration in nutrition: Less than body requirements related to inability to ingest food

Sleep pattern deficit related to postoperative pain, environmental noise

Self-care deficit related to appliances, prostheses, and assistive devices to achieve self-care

From Kim MJ, McFarland GK, McLane AM (eds): Pocket Guide to Nursing Diagnoses. St. Louis, CV Mosby, 1984

| Respiratory Complications

Postoperative respiratory complications are the most frequent cause of death and morbidity in patients having had an anesthetic and surgery. They are the largest single cause of complications after major surgery and the second most common cause of postoperative death in patients more than 60 years of age.

Patients particularly prone to postoperative respiratory complications are those undergoing thoracic and upper abdominal operations who have incisions near the diaphragm. The incidence of postoperative respiratory complications is lower for patients having pelvic surgery and lower still for those having surgeries performed outside the thoracic or abdominal cavities.

A variety of factors increase the potential for respiratory complications. These include preexisting chronic obstructive pulmonary diseases such as chronic bronchitis, emphysema, and chronic asthma; advanced age; obesity; poor nutrition; smoking; prolonged immobilization, and lengthy surgery.

Postoperative pulmonary complications discussed in this section are atelectasis, aspiration, and pneumonia. Pulmonary embolism is presented in the cardiovascular section.

Atelectasis

Regardless of the surgical site or the general anesthetic used, pulmonary function is impaired to some degree postoperatively. Major changes uniformly occur postoperatively in lung volume, pulmonary mechanics, and gas exchange. These changes may lead to significant mismatching of ventilation and perfusion as well as atelectasis, even in the absence of tracheobronchial secretions. Respiratory capacity and function usually return to normal within 12 to 14 days.

Induction of general anesthesia reduces the volume of air remaining in the lung at the end of each expiration. It is the relationship of this volume (the functional residual capacity) to the closing capacity (the volume of the lung where small airways begin to close) that determines if areas of the lung remain open for gas exchange during the ventilatory cycle. Additionally, anesthesia changes the shape and movement of the chest wall, the distribution of ventilation and perfusion within the lungs, and dulls the responsiveness of the respiratory center to carbon dioxide.

Atelectasis, the incomplete expansion of a lung or a portion of it, is the most common postoperative pulmonary complication. In most patients it is partly attributable to the absence of periodic deep breaths. Normally the respiratory pattern of spontaneously breathing adults includes periodic sighs or deep breaths. However, when a person is anesthetized, placed in one position, and ventilated at a constant tidal volume, he does not sigh or take deep breaths. Functional residual capacity decreases, as do lung expansion and gas exchange. Alveoli collapse, and arteriovenous shunting and some degree of hypoxemia occur.

Atelectasis most frequently occurs within 48 hours after surgery and affects 25% of patients having abdominal surgery. Atelectasis is responsible for more than 90% of the febrile episodes that occur during the first 48 hours after surgery. Although all patients have some degree of atelectasis and therefore hypoxemia postoperatively, atelectasis is usually self-limiting and recovery is uneventful.

There are several types of atelectasis, but the type most likely to occur postoperatively is absorption atelectasis. This type is also known as obstructive, reabsorption, or secondary atelectasis and results when secretions or foreign material completely obstruct the airway. Secretions in the bronchi and bronchioles obstruct the airways and prohibit the movement of air into the alveoli. In alveoli distal to the obstruction, soluble gases such as oxygen are absorbed into the bloodstream, and the alveoli collapse. When the alveolar sacs collapse they produce little or no surfactant. Surfactant, which has a short half-life, must be constantly replenished and this requires normal ventilation. Decreased surfactant activity contributes to early airway closure.

Collapsed alveoli are excluded from gaseous exchange. Perfusion to the collapsed alveoli remains unchanged, but a portion of the cardiac output perfuses nonventilating alveoli. There is an increase in venous admixture.

Blood flowing through the pulmonary capillaries that are in contact with the collapsed alveoli does not pick up any oxygen. The result is a perfusion ventilation shunt or a direct right-to-left shunt across the lungs. That is, atelectasis causes a pathological shunting of blood from the right to the left side of the heart. The immediate effect of atelectasis is decreased oxygenation of the blood because desaturated blood enters the systemic circulation. Significant hypoxemia accompanies significant atelectasis, but the patient's respiratory and cardiac reserves determine its clinical significance.

If the respiratory rate increases, excess carbon dioxide is blown off, but the oxygen level remains low. Oxygen takes a longer time to diffuse into the blood stream and attach to the hemoglobin than it does for carbon dioxide to diffuse into the alveoli. Therefore, the patient's respiratory rate increases, but the arterial carbon dioxide level is normal. The arterial pH is normal, and the arterial oxygen level is decreased.

Hypoxemia contributes to the fatigue that surgical patients experience. Additionally, it contributes to the confusion of elderly postoperative patients and to the irritability and discomfort voiced by some postoperative patients.

The postoperative patient is susceptible to atelectasis because of an ineffective cough that causes him to retain secretions. Several factors contribute to an ineffective cough reflex. These include pain; narcotics; position of the incision, especially near the diaphragm; obesity and extreme underweight; advanced age; poor nutrition; uncontrolled preoperative respiratory infections; postoperative respiratory infection; smoking; prolonged immobilization; the supine position, and preexisting respiratory diseases.

Pain makes it difficult to cough effectively, and many narcotics used to relieve pain depress the cough reflex. Thoracic and high abdominal incisions make moving and coughing painful. Additionally, the patient's vital capacity is diminished and alveolar expansion is inadequate due to decreased sighing. Sputum becomes more viscous and tends to gravitate to the dependent area of the lungs. Secretions in the larger airways are an excellent medium for bacterial growth and stasis pneumonia. In fact, pneumonia is almost a certainty if any pulmonary segment is atelectatic for more than 72 hours.

Obese people have a decreased functional residual capacity and increased closing capacity. Futhermore, obesity makes coughing and moving more difficult and also decreases the efficiency of the respiratory muscles. Similarly, underweight persons are at risk for atelectasis because of reduced respiratory muscle mass.

Advanced age increases the risk of postoperative atelectasis because the rib cage becomes less elastic and the lungs lose their recoil. Also, closing capacity increases with age.

Poor nutrition leads to a decrease in gamma globulin and atrophy of the respiratory membranes. These factors increase the potential of infection.

Colds, sore throats, and respiratory infections that are uncontrolled preoperatively lead to atelectasis, as do postoperative respiratory infections. Similarly, smoking, which is associated with retained secretions, contributes to the development of postoperative atelectasis. By interfering with the mucociliary activity that moves sputum from the lower airways to the nose or mouth, smoking impairs the lung's self-cleansing process. Smoking is also believed to increase closing capacity.

Prolonged immobilization, either on the operating table or postoperatively, leads to pooling of secretions in the bronchi as well as to decreased chest expansion. Previously existing respiratory diseases with retained secretions and inadequate alveolar expansion also contribute to atelectasis.

Clinical Manifestations

The signs and symptoms that the patient exhibits depend upon the severity of the atelectasis and the extent of the shunting. In postoperative atelectasis rales in the bases and/or diminished breath sounds are common upon auscultation of the affected part. Similarly, flatness is common on percussion. Symptoms may be absent in mild cases. But as the atelectasis progresses or becomes more widespread, dyspnea, tachypnea, tachycardia, cough, fever, hypotension, and decreased chest expansion on the affected side may occur. In the presence of significant atelectasis, blood gas analysis shows hypoxemia. The patient is weak, anxious, and restless and, as the hypoxemia worsens, he becomes increasingly confused. Hypercapnia and decreased pH may portend respiratory failure.

Preventive Nursing Interventions

1. Identify patients at high risk.
2. Administer pain medication so that the patient can move comfortably, walk, and cough, if he is retaining secretions.
3. Teach and encourage the patient to take deep breaths to maximal inspiratory volume, to hold the inspiration for three seconds, and to repeat the process 3 times per hour while awake. Also teach and encourage the patient to yawn, sigh, and use an incentive spirometer. (See Chapter 3 for specific patient instructions.)
4. Encourage coughing, if the patient has secretions. However, coughing is contraindicated in patients who have had a craniotomy, a hiatal hernia repair, or eye and ear surgery.

    NOTE: The patient's risk factors and hourly progress determine the type and frequency of respiratory exercises. Patients having had a general anesthetic benefit from performing them every hour during the first postoperative day and then every 3 to 4 hours if still inactive.

    Study results indicate that frequent, vigorous, and coached respiratory exercises, with or without devices, is *the* key to decreasing postoperative atelectasis and pneumonia. Encouragement and reinforcement of instruction throughout each postoperative hour is imperative.
5. Suction the patient who has secretions, but is unable to cough effectively.

6. Encourage and assist the patient to turn from side to side.
7. Encourage early ambulation.
8. Position the patient properly, that is, assist him to an upright or semiupright position. The weight of the abdomen against the diaphragm restricts its movement. Proper positioning allows the lungs to expand fully.

Therapy

Treatment of atelectasis involves measures to clear the airway. Chest percussion, coughing, or nasotracheal suction may be used. For patients with severe chronic obstructive pulmonary disease, bronchodilators and mucolytic agents via nebulizer may be helpful. If a major airway is obstructed and contributing to atelectasis, intrabronchial suction via bronchoscopy may be required.

Some physicians advocate intermittent continuous positive airway pressure (CPAP) by face mask for treating atelectasis that is unresponsive to routine therapy in alert and spontaneously breathing patients. CPAP is the application of positive pressure throughout the respiratory cycle. By preventing airway pressure from returning to zero, CPAP helps reopen collapsed alveoli and prevents small airway closure at the end of respiration. Although CPAP requires no effort from the patient and is not painful, it remains controversial.

Pneumonia

Pneumonia is an inflammatory response in which cellular material replaces alveolar gas. Pneumonia can be viral or bacterial in etiology, but approximately half of postoperative pulmonary infections are caused by gram-negative bacilli. While gram-negative bacteria colonize the oropharynx in only 20% of normal persons, colonization is common after major surgery due to impaired oropharyngeal mechanisms.

Postoperative pneumonia develops a few days after surgery. Predisposing factors include aspiration; infection; copious secretions; atelectasis; prolonged immobilization; dehydration, and disruption of normal host defenses. Certain host defenses normally minimize a patient's susceptibility to pneumonia. These defenses are the cough reflex, the mucociliary system, and activity of alveolar macrophages.

Postoperatively these defenses are weak. The cough reflex may not effectively clear the bronchial tree. The mucociliary transport mechanism may be damaged by endotracheal intubation. Factors such as the administration of oxygen and corticosteroids, pulmonary edema, and aspiration compromise the functional ability of the alveolar macrophages. Additionally, squamous metaplasia and loss of ciliary coordination impede antibacterial defenses.

Clinical Manifestations

Clinical manifestations of postoperative pneumonia depend upon its location and extent. Subjective findings include dyspnea; tachypnea; pleuritic chest pain; fever; chills; hemoptysis, and a cough that produces rusty or purulent sputum. Objective findings include fever; hypoxemia; percussion dullness; coarse inspiratory rales, and decreased breath sounds over the involved area. A chest x-ray shows localized parenchymal consolidation.

Preventive Nursing Interventions

1. Identify patients at risk.
2. Prevent aspiration and regurgitation through proper positioning.
3. Assist and encourage the patient to take deep breaths to maximal inspiratory volume, that is, to yawn, sigh, and use an incentive spirometer.
4. Assist the patient to cough and to turn from side to side.
5. Encourage early ambulation.
6. Maintain adequate hydration.
7. Suction patients who are unable to clear secretions.

Therapy

The treatment goal is to clear the patient's airway and maintain its patency. Nursing interventions that facilitate attainment of this goal include improving ventilation; providing adequate pain medication so that the patient can move and cough; keeping him adequately hydrated; providing chest percussion (or vibration) and postural drainage, and planning the patient's care so that he is able to conserve his energy. Medically, antibiotics are ordered after the causative organism is identified. A sputum specimen is obtained directly from the trachea, usually by endotracheal suctioning.

Aspiration

Aspiration generally refers to the inhalation into the tracheobronchial system of gastric contents, food, water, or blood. Postoperatively, aspiration is most often a result of regurgitation, a passive process unlike vomiting. Regurgitation is frequently "silent" in patients with altered or depressed mental states.

Normally, the gastroesophageal and pharyngeal sphincters prevent aspiration, but a variety of factors in the intra- and postoperative periods predispose a patient to aspiration. These factors include the depression of the central nervous system via drugs that interfere with such protective mechanisms as the cough and gag reflexes, and insertion of nasogastric and endotracheal tubes. A nasogastric tube predisposes a patient to aspiration because the tube renders both the upper and lower esophageal sphincters at least partially incompetent. If the tube is not expertly placed and properly functioning, regurgitation and aspiration are likely to occur. Furthermore, suction via a nasogastric tube does not guarantee complete gastric emptying.

Grossly evident aspiration and subsequent pneumonia are associated with a 50% mortality rate. Massive aspiration of gastric contents is associated with a 70% to 90% mortality rate.

Aspiration of gastric contents causes chemical irritation or pneumonitis.

This results in local edema, inflammation, and destruction of the mucosa of the tracheobronchial tree. These changes increase the risk of secondary infection. The severity of the response depends upon the patient's physiologic status, as well as on the quantity and acidity of the aspirant, the frequency of aspiration, and the distribution of the aspirate.

With a pH of 2.5 or less, gastric contents are very acidic and when aspirated, cause a typically severe response. Aspiration of gastric contents with a pH between 1.5 and 2.5 causes a progressively severe response. Aspiration of gastric contents with a pH less than 1.5 causes little additional damage, but the outcome is uniformly fatal.

The severity of the reaction has been related to the volume of gastric juice aspirated. Volumes of 50 ml with a pH of 2.4 cause overwhelming damage. Fasting patients being prepared for surgery typically have at least 50 ml of fluid in their stomachs and in fasting patients, the pH is 1.5 to 2.4.

Clinical Manifestations

Those seen depend upon the severity of the aspiration. Atelectatic areas typically appear soon after aspiration and become extensive within 2 minutes. Respiratory distress begins within 1 minute to 60 minutes after gastric acid aspiration. Tachypnea, dyspnea, cough, and bronchospasm follow reflex airway closure. Wheezes, rhonchi, and rales are heard in more than one third of patients, and depending upon the amount of ventilation-perfusion defect, cyanosis may develop.

In aspiration, alveolar cells are destroyed, together with a subsequent loss of surfactant. Additionally, within the first few hours after aspiration, pulmonary capillary cells and the endothelial lining are destroyed. Capillary permeability increases and the alveoli and bronchi become flooded with fluid. Pulmonary edema ensues and creates areas of hypoventilation and shunting with severe hypoxemia. The surfactant destruction facilitates alveolar collapse and further atelectasis. The result is a classic example of noncardiac pulmonary edema. Findings resemble those of adult respiratory distress syndrome.

The amount of fluid lost from the intravascular compartment into the lungs determines subsequent pulmonary and cardiac responses. If a massive amount of fluid is lost, the secretions are pink and frothy. Rales are unilateral or bilateral, and chest x-ray shows infiltrates. Although the exact location of the infiltrates depends on the patient's position when he aspirated, the basilar segments are most often affected. The infiltrates develop progressively and are fully demarcated within 24 to 36 hours after aspiration.

The massive fluid shift that occurs causes hypovolemia. Arterial hypotension may occur after aspiration and up to 25% of patients who aspirate develop shock. Similarly, the hematocrit rises due to hemoconcentration. Excessive fluid and colloid are lost into the injured lung.

Metabolic acidosis also develops in aspiration pneumonia. Hypoxemia and poor peripheral perfusion with a subsequent accumulation of lactate ion are responsible for this imbalance.

Preventive Nursing Interventions
1. Identify patients at risk.
2. Assess patients closely for impaired level of consciousness after giving central nervous system depressants.
3. Position unconscious patients on the right side with the head tilted down, unless contraindicated.
4. Suction the pharynx and trachea as necessary.
5. Position patients with nasogastric tubes in a semi-Fowler's position unless contraindicated.
6. Maintain the patency and proper functioning of nasogastric tubes.
7. Position patients with hiatal hernia in a semi-Fowler's position.
8. Administer cimetidine and ranitidine as ordered. These are used to decrease gastric acidity and to some extent volume. Also, metoclopramide (Reglan) is being tested for use with at-risk patients. It increases gastric emptying and more importantly, is said to increase gastroesophageal sphincter tone.

Therapy

The treatment of aspiration depends upon the extent of the damage. Measures include reestablishing and maintaining a patent airway; preventing future damage; performing endotracheal suctioning; reducing hypoxemia and correcting hypovolemia, and performing bronchoscopy to remove solid matter.

Evaluation

The patient develops no clinically significant postoperative respiratory complications.

Cardiovascular Complications

Postoperative complications involving the cardiovascular system include shock, deep vein thrombosis, and embolism. Although pulmonary embolism is a respiratory complication, it is included in this section because most pulmonary emboli arise from deep venous thrombosis of the lower extremities.

Shock

Circulatory impairment that diminishes the normal metabolic processes of cells characterizes the complex clinical syndrome known as shock. Inadequate tissue perfusion and decreased tissue oxygenation cause a host of physiologic responses.

Two types of shock for which the postoperative patient is at risk are hypovolemic and septic. In these two types, just as in cardiogenic and neurogenic shock, the primary pathophysiological problem occurs in the microcirculation at the capillary level.

Hypovolemic Shock

Although the most common cause of hypovolemic shock in the postoperative patient is hemorrhage, hypovolemic shock can also result from severe dehydration and the sequestration of fluid. In shock due to decreased blood volume, the blood volume is inadequate to fill the circulatory system. That is, the size of the intravascular compartment is increased in relation to the intravascular blood volume.

A reduced intravascular volume causes decreased venous return. In turn, the filling pressure of the ventricles, stroke volume, cardiac output, and blood pressure all decrease. The result is decreased tissue perfusion with less nutrients and oxygen delivered to the cells.

A decrease in venous return and cardiac output causes the pressure-sensitive baroreceptors in the aortic arch and carotid bodies to initiate the release of norepinephrine and epinephrine. The output of these catecholamines, which is 10 to 50 times normal, causes sympathetic stimulation. The compensatory mechanisms that occur, such as tachycardia, increased myocardial contractility, and arteriolar vasoconstriction, help maintain cardiac output until about 20% of the circulating volume is lost. If the hemorrhage continues, the cells become deprived of oxygen, organs begin to dysfunction, and cellular damage and failure occur.

Vasoconstriction shunts up to 70% of cardiac output to the brain, while decreasing blood flow to the kidneys, liver, bowel, and skin. Because vasoconstriction preserves cerebral perfusion, restlessness and confusion indicate more severe shock.

Decreasing blood flow to the kidneys causes less fluid to be filtered and renal function is disturbed. In response to the decreasing blood flow and reduced circulating volume, the kidneys release renin, which in turn stimulates the release of angiotensin. Angiotensin is a very potent vasoconstrictor and stimulates aldosterone. The latter enhances retention of sodium and excretion of potassium, thus contributing to fluid retention while renal function is decreasing.

Stagnation of circulation in the capillaries and small vessels and tissue hypoxia cause the body to turn to anaerobic metabolism. Lactic acid accumulates, which causes intracellular acidity. The result is metabolic acidosis and irreversible shock.

Clinical Manifestations

The signs and symptoms of shock depend upon its stage, that is, early, middle, or late (Table 8-1). In early shock the body's compensatory mechanisms maintain arterial blood pressure and cardiac output. The patient is oriented to person, place, and time. In the middle stage of shock, arterial blood pressure and cardiac output are decreased. The patient is oriented, but may slur his words. In late shock, the compensatory mechanisms are nonexistent, and multiple organ failure is imminent.

Table 8-1
Clinical Picture Exhibited by Patient
According to Degree of Shock

	Early	Middle	Late
Sensorium	Oriented to time, place, person	Remains oriented; words slurred	Disoriented
Pulse	Rate, 110–120 Quality, full to decreased	Rate, 120–150 Quality, decreased and variable	Rate, greater than 150 Quality, weak
Blood pressure	Normal to low (10%–20% decrease but may be slightly increased as compensatory mechanism)	Decreased 40–50 mm Hg below normal (20%–40% decrease)	Systolic less than 80 Diastolic may not be heard
Urinary output	30–50 ml/hr	20–35 ml/hr	Less than 20 ml/hr
Color	Pale	Pale	Mottled
Capillary refill	Circulation return slightly slowed	Circulation return slowed	Circulation return very slowed; skin pale both before and after Large differences between rectal and big toe temperature

From Kenner C, Guzzetta C, Dossey B: Critical Care Nursing: Body-Mind-Spirit, p 770. Boston, Little, Brown & Co, 1981

Preventive Nursing Interventions

1. Identify patients at risk.
2. Continually reassess patients at risk.
3. Monitor and record vital signs, looking for increasing pulse and decreasing blood pressure. Trends are more important than individual values.
4. Monitor the patient's fluid balance and note insensible losses such as profuse perspiration and excessive wound drainage. Keep accurate intake and output records, measure and record urine specific gravity.
5. Weigh the patient daily, at the same time, on the same scale, with the same amount of clothing and linen, before eating, and after voiding.
6. Assess the color, temperature, turgor, and moistness of the patient's skin and mucous membranes. Cyanosis is not only a late, but also an unreliable, sign of inadequate tissue perfusion.
7. Assess the patient's level of consciousness. Any change in the

patient's level of consciousness should alert the nurse to decreasing cerebral perfusion.

Therapy

When treating the patient in hypovolemic shock the goal is to restore cellular perfusion as soon as possible. Achieving this goal hinges upon rapidly restoring circulating intravascular volume and cardiac output, while treating the underlying problem.

Placing the patient flat in bed enhances cardiac and cerebral circulation, and slightly elevating the legs promotes venous return and cardiac output. The patient can be turned from side to side, but should not be placed in Trendelenburg position because it impedes respiratory efforts.

Oxygen is administered via mask or cannula. The patient is covered with a light blanket to conserve energy.

Large-bore intravenous catheters are inserted to facilitate rapid volume replacement. Crystalloid solutions such as Lactated Ringer's are infused. Lactated Ringer's is frequently the solution of choice for immediate replacement because it closely resembles plasma electrolytes. Although rarely associated with adverse reactions, Lactated Ringer's is contraindicated in patients with liver failure because they are unable to metabolize lactate.

Blood pressure and pulse rate are monitored as indices of perfusion. If the administration of intravenous crystalloid solutions does not reverse the hypovolemia, a colloid such as normal human serum albumin may be administered.

Blood is administered when acute anemia reaches the point of critical hemodilution. Warming refrigerated blood prior to administration prevents hypothermia and additional vasoconstriction. Arterial blood gas values, blood chemistries, and complete blood counts are used to evaluate the effectiveness of therapy.

A urinary output of less than 30 ml per hour indicates decreased renal perfusion. Oliguria despite adequate hydration necessitates immediate interventions to prevent renal shutdown. Mannitol is given because its osmotic pull draws fluid into the intravascular space. Furosemide (Lasix) may be ordered, if the mannitol is ineffective.

Restoring cellular perfusion usually alleviates metabolic acidosis; sodium bicarbonate is administered if it persists. Sodium bicarbonate not only improves acid-base balance, but also enhances the function of other medications and body organs. If shock still persists, dopamine hydrochloride (Inotropin) may be needed to increase blood pressure and improve cardiac output.

Throughout the treatment of hypovolemic shock, the nurse evaluates the patient's response to therapy. She monitors his vital functions, including level of consciousness, pulse rate, blood pressure, and urine output, including specific gravity. She maintains a calm and confident attitude and reassures the patient and his family. She alleviates their anxiety and fears and explains the plan of care. Additionally, she facilitates visits from family members.

Septic Shock

Septic shock is a type of distributive shock. Unlike hypovolemic shock in which blood volume is decreased, in septic shock blood is abnormally distributed in the circulatory network. This alteration leads to decreased peripheral resistance and increased vascular capacity. Just as in hypovolemic shock, however, the primary problem is inadequate tissue perfusion and decreased tissue oxygenation.

A variety of organisms, including viruses, fungi, and both gram-positive and gram-negative bacteria, cause septic shock. However, gram-negative bacteria are the most prevalent, accounting for 75% of all cases of septic shock. Furthermore, approximately 70% of all cases of gram-negative septicemia are the result of nosocomial or hospital acquired infection. The incidence of shock in patients with gram-negative septicemia is 40%, and the mortality rate for patients who develop shock is at least 40%. In decreasing order of frequency, the gram-negative bacteria responsible for septic shock are *Escherichia coli, Klebsiella pneumoniae, Enterobacter, Proteus,* and *Pseudomonas.*

Septic shock occurs most commonly in patients with altered host defenses and in whom medical and/or surgical treatments have interrupted normal defenses. Specific patients at high risk for septic shock include:

1. Those more than 65 years of age
2. Those with diabetes
3. Those who have undergone urological procedures such as cystoscopies, catheterizations, and transurethral resections. The genitourinary tract is the primary source of microorganisms causing septic shock
4. Those having surgery
5. Those with chronic or debilitating diseases
6. Those with central venous lines

Gram-negative bacteria contain a lipopolysaccharide-protein complex within their cell walls. When the immune system destroys the bacteria, this complex, called endotoxin, is released. The body's reaction to endotoxin causes septic shock. Known to activate the complement, coagulation, fibrinolytic, and kinin systems, endotoxin initiates many biochemical changes that cause disastrous effects.

While septic shock due to gram-negative bacteria is frequently called endotoxic shock, not all septic shock is endotoxic shock. However, the shock caused by gram-negative bacteria is more virulent than that caused by other organisms. Thus, the clinical course described is limited to that caused by gram-negative organisms.

Endotoxin can cause two clinical stages. The first is called hyperdynamic shock, the second, hypodynamic shock.

In hyperdynamic, "high output," or warm shock, the body reacts to the causative organism. Endotoxin is released from the bacterial cell wall into the tissues. It directly damages them, and alters cellular metabolism. Endotoxin impairs the ability of the cells to use oxygen and other nutrients. Additionally, blood is shunted away from the nutritional capillaries. Because endotoxin disturbs the biochemical activity of the cells, cellular function is impaired.

Vasoactive substances such as bradykinin are released from damaged cells. Because these substances cause both the arteriolar and venous vascular beds to dilate, blood pressure and peripheral resistance fall. This venous pooling not only decreases venous return, but also reduces ventricular filling pressures. The arteriovenous shunting and the vasodilation decrease peripheral resistance. Although blood pressure is decreased, cardiac output may be normal or high because of the ease with which the heart can pump against low pressure and low resistance. The duration of the hyperdynamic stage of septic shock varies significantly. It may last 30 minutes to 16 hours.

Progression of the shock state leads to hypodynamic, "low output," or cold shock. In this stage the patient develops the "typical" signs and symptoms of shock. Endotoxin causes the release of other such vasoactive substances as histamine. By increasing capillary permeability and allowing plasma to leak from the intravascular space, histamine causes a relative hypovolemia.

The compensatory mechanisms initiated by the catecholamines are insufficient, however. Thus, venous return and ventricular filling pressures are reduced. These events potentiate decreased stroke volume, decreased cardiac output, and decreased blood pressure.

Vasoconstriction due to high levels of catecholamines and angiotensin is marked. Oxygen deprivation and intracellular acidosis increase, accelerating cell death. Organ failure begins. Coronary and hepatic blood flow decreases as does renal function. Multiple organ dysfunction is the cause of death.

Clinical Manifestations

The clinical manifestations of gram-negative septic shock depend upon just when in the syndrome the patient is observed and also upon his prior physical condition. Presenting signs and symptoms in the hyperdynamic stage include fever and chills; warm, dry skin that is flushed; slight alteration in mental status; and increased pulse and respiratory rates. Blood pressure is moderately decreased, and urinary output is decreased while specific gravity is increased. However, the older and the sicker the patient, the less likely he is to manifest these signs and symptoms. For example, fever is unlikely to occur in the elderly.

In the hypodynamic stage chills and fever may be present. Skin is pale, moist, and cold; level of consciousness is markedly decreased, and both pulse and respiratory rates are significantly increased. Blood pressure and urinary output are sharply decreased. Adult respiratory distress syndrome and disseminated intravascular coagulation occur late in the hypodynamic stage.

Preventive Nursing Interventions

1. Identify patients at risk for septic shock.
2. Monitor and record the patient's vital signs carefully, being alert to signs and symptoms of systemic infection.

3. Use optimal aseptic technique when inserting all intracirculatory system catheters.
4. Cover arterial lines, CVP, and Swan-Ganz insertion sites with sterile dressings.
5. Observe intracirculatory insertion sites for signs and symptoms of inflammation.
6. Review laboratory data, monitoring white blood cell and differential counts.
7. Assess the patient's level of consciousness for alterations.
8. Use indwelling urinary catheters only when absolutely necessary.
9. Minimize urethral trauma by using the smallest catheter possible that ensures unobstructed drainage.
10. Use aseptic technique and sterile equipment when inserting a urinary catheter.
11. Limit the handling and care of catheters to staff who aseptically insert and maintain them.
12. Secure the catheter properly to avoid movement and urethral irritation.
13. Wash hands immediately before and after manipulation of the urinary catheter site or closed drainage bag.
14. Disconnect the catheter and drainage tube only if the catheter is to be irrigated.
15. Irrigate the catheter only to prevent or treat an obstruction.
16. Disinfect the catheter-tubing junction before disconnection.
17. Obtain specimens of fresh urine from the aspiration port.
18. Maintain unobstructed urinary flow.
19. Make sure the tubing is neither tangled nor kinked.
20. Do not allow urine to stand in the tubing.
21. Empty the collection bag at least every 8 hours, more frequently if needed.
22. Make sure each patient with an indwelling urinary catheter has his own collecting container.
23. Never allow the drainage spigot to touch the nonsterile collecting container.
24. Keep the drainage bag below the level of the patient's bladder at all times.
25. Never allow the drainage bag to touch the floor.

Therapy

The survival of the patient in gram-negative septic shock depends upon early recognition and prompt, appropriate intervention. The patient in gram-negative septic shock has the best chance of surviving when treated in the hyperdynamic stage. In the hypodynamic stage, multisystem organ failure is common despite aggressive resuscitation.

In the hyperdynamic stage, rapid administration of intravenous fluids, together with removal or drainage of the source of sepsis, may prevent the progression of shock. Depending upon the patient's condition, other interventions may be necessary. These include the administration of oxygen, the correction of metabolic acidosis, and the administration of antibiotics and other appropriate pharmacologic agents.

Intravenous fluids are rapidly, but cautiously, administered to correct intravascular volume deficit. If adequate tissue perfusion does not correct the metabolic acidosis, intravenous sodium bicarbonate is given. Similarly, if volume replacement does not restore perfusion, sympathomimetic amines such as dopamine hydrochloride (Intropin) and dobutamine (Dobutrex) are administered. The efficacy of corticosteroids in the treatment of gram-negative septic shock remains controversial.

As soon as specimens have been collected for culture and sensitivity, broad-spectrum antibiotic coverage is begun, usually with a cephalosporin plus an aminoglycoside. The therapy becomes organism specific when culture results are available.

Throughout therapy, the nurse monitors the patient's response to interventions. Just as for the patient in hypovolemic shock, she reassures him and calms his fears and those of his family.

Evaluation

The patient is hemodynamically stable.

Deep Venous Thrombosis

Deep venous thrombosis occurs in the pelvic veins or in the deep veins of the lower extremities. Its incidence, which varies between 10% and 40%, is related to the complexity of surgery or severity of illness. Specific surgeries and their associated incidences of deep venous thrombosis are as follows: 51% after retropubic prostatectomy; 74% after fractured hip, and 14% to 33% after general abdominal or thoracic surgery.[1]

The three major factors related to the formation of deep vein thrombosis are venous stasis, injury to the intimal layer of the vein wall, and hypercoagulability. These three factors are known as Virchow's triad, and one or more of them may produce thrombus.

Venous stasis results from a combination of factors. Some are inherent in venous circulation, while others are contributing factors. The venous system has no intrinsic force to move blood through it. Therefore, venous flow is almost totally dependent upon the action of voluntary muscles and the competence of one-way valves. Inactive muscles or incompetent valves result in venous dilation and stasis. Sluggish peripheral circulation due to dehydration, shock, or congestive heart failure also causes venous stasis. Other factors that contribute to stasis and thrombus formation are prolonged bed rest; immobilization; varicose veins; obesity; cigarette smoking; advanced age, and major surgical procedures.

The second major factor of Virchow's triad is damage to the intimal layer of the vein wall. Damage alters the epithelial lining, impairing the fibrinolytic activity that prevents thrombus formation. Cell nutrients leak into the vessel, and platelets aggregate at the site of the damage. Fibrin traps some of the platelets, together with the red blood cells and granular leukocytes. This aggregation combined with low flow of the venous system precipitates thrombus formation.

The third factor of Virchow's triad is hypercoagulability. Instrumentation or surgery stimulates the coagulation cascade causing hypercoagulability. Other conditions that result in hypercoagulability are dehydration; malignancy; the use of oral contraceptives, and a deficiency of antithrombin III. Antithrombin III, a circulating protein, inactivates thrombin and other clotting factors. Thus, a deficiency can lead to a proliferation of thrombin and other clotting factors, and to an increased coagulability of blood.

Two mechanisms may result in the formation of a fibrin clot, the extrinsic and the intrinsic pathways. While trauma to the vessel or tissue surrounding the vessel initiates the former, the latter begins within the blood itself. Both pathways include a series of blood clotting factors that initiate a chain of events when activated. Tissue factor, a proteolytic enzyme, and tissue phospholipids activate the extrinsic pathway. Contact between factor XII and platelets with the collagen in the vessel wall activate the intrinsic pathway.

The nature of flow in the vessels affects the composition of a thrombus. Fibrin is a major component of red thrombi, which have cellular elements distributed evenly throughout. White thrombi are composed of platelet deposits overlaid with fibrin and red and white cells. While red thrombi most frequently occur in veins, white thrombi occur secondary to abnormal vascular surfaces. Thus, anticoagulants readily prevent red thrombi, while drugs that suppress platelet function prevent white thrombi.

Most venous thrombi are thought to form in the sinuses of the venous valves and may extend into the adjacent vein. The thrombi grow in the direction of blood flow. A thrombus slows the flow and occludes part of the vessel. Then, the thrombus grows in both directions. When a clot obstructs the blood flow or when an inflammatory process ensues in the contiguous vein, signs and symptoms become clinically evident. However, 50% or more of venous thrombi escape clinical detection.

Deep vein thrombosis usually develops 7 to 10 days after surgery. Patients at increased risk are those with a history of thromboembolism; pulmonary embolism; varicose veins; blood disorders associated with hypercoagulability such as polycythemia; cardiac diseases such as myocardial infarction and congestive failure; neoplasms, especially adenocarcinoma of the gastrointestinal tract; traumatic injury, and estrogen therapy. Other patients at risk are women over 30 years of age using oral contraceptives; the obese; the immobilized; the elderly; postoperative patients with infections, and those undergoing abdominal or pelvic surgery, a splenectomy, or orthopedic procedures on the leg.

If left untreated, a deep vein thrombus can become an embolus. Blood flow over a formed thrombus may detach all or part of it from the vessel wall. A free thrombus is an embolus that circulates until it meets resistance.

Venous thrombi in the deep veins of the calf rarely embolize to the lungs, and only those emboli above the knee are considered sources of pulmonary emboli. However, 20% of calf vein thrombi extend into major leg veins. This extension, which can occur in minutes, is an embolic potential because the caliber of the veins above the knee is sufficiently large to allow the formation of dangerously large thrombi. More than 15% of the calf vein thrombi migrate upward. An estimated 50% of deep venous thrombi in the iliofemoral venous systems embolize to the lungs. Approximately 10% are fatal.

Clinical Manifestations

The patient may be asymptomatic unless the thrombus completely obstructs venous blood flow. Phlebothrombosis, thrombus formation without inflammation of the vein wall, is the most common type of deep vein thrombosis in immobilized and/or obese patients and in those who have undergone surgery.

The majority of calf vein thrombi are asymptomatic. When present, symptoms of calf vein thrombi include swelling, pain, and tenderness in the affected calf muscle. This may be accompanied by a feeling of warmth or heaviness. Malaise and fever (with or without chills) may also occur. When the femoral and iliac veins are involved, symptoms in the acute phase are more likely. They include tenderness over those veins, swelling, and cyanosis of the skin.

Diagnosis of deep vein thrombosis from signs and symptoms alone is rare because many other conditions cause similar sign and symptoms. In fact, more than 59% of patients with deep vein thrombosis confirmed by diagnostic tests do not exhibit characteristic signs and symptoms. A positive Homan's sign, calf pain upon dorsiflexion of the foot, does not definitely indicate deep vein thrombosis because rupture of the plantar muscle and superficial phlebitis can also cause calf pain upon dorsiflexion.

Noninvasive diagnostic tests have proved to be the most useful in detecting deep vein thrombosis. Doppler ultrasonography and impedance plethysmography are most commonly performed. The incidence of false-positives is extraordinarily low, and the accuracy rate of these two tests together is about 95%.

In Doppler ultrasonography ultrahigh-frequency sound waves are transmitted through the skin. Circulating red blood cells reflect these sound waves at frequencies that vary with the rate of blood flow through the vessel. Doppler ultrasonography is highly sensitive to popliteal, femoral, or iliac vein thrombosis but insensitive to calf vein thrombosis.

In impedance plethysmography blood volume changes in the calves cause changes in electrical resistance of the calves. These changes are recorded on an ECG strip. While extremely sensitive to symptomatic proximal vein thrombi, impedance plethysmography is insensitive to calf vein clots.

The 125-I-labeled fibrinogen scan is another test used in diagnosing deep vein thrombosis. It is extremely sensitive to calf vein thrombi, but insensitive to clots in the pelvic veins. 125-I-labeled fibrinogen is injected into the venous system. An isotope detector is used to measure increases in surface radioactivity that represent uptake by the thrombi.

The reference standard for diagnosing deep venous thrombosis is venography. An invasive procedure that involves the injection of a contrast medium into the patient's bloodstream, venography is both the most definitive diagnostic test and also the most risky. Some authorities believe that Doppler ultrasonography, impedance plethysmography, and/or leg scanning may eliminate the need for venography.

Preventive Nursing Interventions

1. Identify patients at high risk for deep vein thrombosis preoperatively.
2. Encourage early ambulation, unless contraindicated.
3. Teach and encourage the patient to dorsiflex his feet for 5 minutes every hour.
4. Perform passive range of motion exercises for a bedridden patient.
5. Elevate the legs 10 to 15 degrees above the horizontal plane of the body. This results in a 30% increase in blood flow. The legs can be elevated by raising the foot of the bed or by placing pillows under their entire length. Avoid using the knee gatch and elevating the patient's knees with pillows. These measures can obstruct venous blood flow.
6. Preoperatively teach and encourage the patient to deep breathe postoperatively. Deep breathing not only ventilates the lungs, but also promotes venous return. (See Chapter 3 for specific patient instructions.)
7. Teach the patient to avoid standing or sitting in one place for a long time and to avoid crossing his legs when sitting. Prolonged standing and sitting, as well as crossing the legs, decrease venous flow and contribute to stasis.
8. Teach the patient to place his feet flat on the floor when sitting at the edge of the bed and to avoid dangling his legs over the edge of the bed. This alleviates pressure on the popliteal area.
9. Avoid rubbing or massaging the calves of the legs, and teach the patient and his family not to do so. Rubbing may fragment the clot, causing an embolus.
10. Apply, as ordered, antiembolism stockings or elastic bandages that uniformly distribute pressure. Make sure the stockings fit. Elastic support bandages must not be too tight at the proximal end or too loose at the distal end. Intermittent pneumatic compression stockings may be ordered for selected patients. These include long-term bedridden patients, those in whom

anticoagulant therapy is either contraindicated, that is, neurosurgical patients, or those in whom it has been found to be ineffective, that is, prostatecomy patients. Intermittent pneumatic compression stockings have not been found to decrease femoral vein thrombosis or pulmonary embolism.

NOTE: Study results indicate that neither antiembolism stockings alone nor leg elevation alone reduce the frequency of postoperative deep vein thrombosis by more than one third. Thus, a combination of these measures, together with active or passive leg exercises, is essential.[2]

11.   Assess the patient regularly. Check his legs for swelling, asymmetric size, inflammation, pain, deep muscle or generalized tenderness, cyanosis, and venous distention. Also monitor his temperature for low-grade fever. All are associated with thrombophlebitis.

12.   Monitor the patient's fluid balance. Both over and underhydration can decrease venous return and cause venous stasis in the legs.

13.   Avoid inserting I.V. catheters in legs and feet. This increases the risk of thrombus formation.

14.   Encourage the patient to stop smoking. By constricting the veins, nicotine decreases venous blood flow.

15.   If the patient is obese,encourage weight reduction after discharge. Extra pounds increase pressure on the veins in the legs.

16.   Administer low-dose heparin or dextran as ordered to prevent clotting. Low-dose heparin inhibits the formation of thrombin but has little effect on clotting studies. Contraindications to low-dose heparin are known bleeding disorders, prostatectomy, cerebral or ophthalmic surgery, extensive orthopedic procedures, and malignant hyperthermia. The major complication of low-dose heparin is wound hematoma.

Dextran, a glucose polymer, has antithrombotic properties. Although it expands blood volume, decreases blood viscosity, and reduces platelet reactivity, its effectiveness in preventing deep vein thrombosis in surgical patients is controversial. Its primary side-effect is volume overload and resulting cardiac failure. It is also associated with anaphylaxis and in higher doses increases bleeding time.

Therapy

Once a thrombus has formed, treatment is the highest priority. Treatment involves both pharmacologic and nonpharmacologic intervention. Typically, heparin and warfarin (Coumadin) are used to prevent further clot formation and extension of the thrombus, and to minimize the risk of pulmonary embolism. Analgesics are ordered to relieve pain.

Heparin is the first drug given, because it achieves peak effect within minutes of administration. It increases the activity of antithrombin III, thus prolonging the clotting times. Additionally, it prevents the conversion of prothrombin to thrombin, which in turn blocks the conversion of fibrinogen to fibrin. In the majority of patients heparin halts the thrombotic process and limits extension of the clot. Within 8 to 10 days the clot dissolves or is incorporated into the vein wall. Heparin therapy is maintained for 7 to 14 days.

Warfarin sodium prevents vitamin K modification of clotting factors II (prothrombin), VII, IX, and X, all of which are formed in the liver. However, because warfarin does not act upon already formed clotting factors, it does not become effective until all active circulating clotting factors have been depleted. The depletion takes about 4 to 7 days from the start of therapy. Because of its delayed action, warfarin is usually administered simultaneously with heparin, either at the beginning or toward the end of heparin therapy. Once the desired level of anticoagulation has been achieved, the heparin is discontinued, and the patient is maintained on warfarin. The location of the thrombus and the incidence of pulmonary embolism determine the duration of the warfarin therapy.

Stool softeners are ordered to eliminate straining at stool. The Valsalva maneuver, forcible exhalation against a closed glottis, increases intrathoracic pressure and interferes with venous return. When air is exhaled, the increased intrathoracic pressure falls, resulting in a sudden increase in venous return to the heart. These sudden pressure changes can dislodge a thrombus. Additionally, the patient is instructed not to strain when having a bowel movement.

Symptomatic treatment involves bed rest, elevation of the affected leg, and careful handling of the affected leg. Bed rest, with the foot of the bed elevated 10 to 15 degrees, promotes venous return and decreases swelling. If the foot of the bed is elevated, the head of the bed should be flat to prevent inguinal congestion. If the leg is elevated on pillows, they must be placed under the entire length of the affected leg to prevent compression of the popliteal vein.

The duration of bed rest is controversial, but continues as long as the patient has signs and symptoms. Usually 7 days after the onset of the thrombus its tail will be attached to the vessel wall.

The affected leg is handled carefully and gently. Trauma and sudden movement of the leg may cause a clot to dislodge.

The circulation, motor, and neurologic function in each foot is checked and compared to the other foot each shift. Additionally, the circumference of each leg is measured and recorded daily.

An antiembolic stocking or elastic support bandage is applied to the unaffected leg. Antiembolic stockings and elastic support bandages promote venous return and decrease stasis. By compressing the superficial veins, they direct the blood flow to the deep veins. Antiembolism stockings and elastic support bandages are not generally applied to the affected leg during the acute phase, but may be ordered when the patient starts to walk. However, when wrapped, the affected leg is not wrapped above the knee because this puts pressure on the popliteal vein, which exacerbates venous stasis. The leg should be elevated before wrapping and wrapped from the toes up. Wrapping from the calf down increases venous engorgement. The stocking or bandage is worn continuously but is removed and reapplied at least once per shift.

Surgery is rarely used in the treatment of deep vein thrombosis. However, if the thrombus is very fresh and located in large vessel, a thrombectomy may be performed. Additionally, if a patient has a history of deep vein thrombosis and anticoagulant therapy is contraindicated, vena caval surgery, that is, insertion of an umbrella, filter, or clip, may be performed to intercept migrating thrombi. This surgery may also be performed for patients who have not benefited from anticoagulant therapy.

Pulmonary Embolism

Pulmonary embolism is the most serious complication of deep vein thrombosis. However, less than 50% of patients with documented pulmonary emboli have clinically apparent thrombophlebitis. Untreated pulmonary embolism is associated with a 30% mortality rate, treated pulmonary embolism, with an 8% to 9% mortality rate. Factors predisposing a patient to pulmonary embolism are those predisposing a patient to thromboembolism.

More than 90% of all pulmonary emboli emanate from thrombi within the deep veins of the thigh or pelvis. The tail of a thrombus breaks loose and becomes an embolus, traveling through the veins to the right side of the heart. The pumping action of the heart breaks the embolus into many little pieces. A clot that travels to the lungs can be small enough to cause no symptoms or large enough to block off the pulmonary artery, causing immediate death. Eighty percent of the deaths resulting from pulmonary embolism occur within two hours of a massive embolization, and the overall mortality rate is 38%.

In the lungs, the embolus decreases the size of the pulmonary vascular bed and increases pulmonary vascular resistance. However, because of the pulmonary vasculature's large reserve capacity, more than 50% of pulmonary arterial circulation must be lost before signs of pulmonary hypotension develop. If an embolus occludes more than 50% of the pulmonary circulation, work load on the right heart increases. Right ventricular failure and decreased cardiac output ensue.

Obstruction of pulmonary blood flow creates an area of alveolar dead space that continues to be ventilated but not perfused. Right-to-left intrapulmonary shunting occurs and accounts for most of the hypoxemia observed in patients. However, the magnitude of the shunting does not correlate with the percentage of the pulmonary vascular bed embolized. Terminal airway constriction follows obstruction and decreases the amount of dead space. Additionally, the nonperfused alveoli slowly lose surfactant. Bronchoconstriction may be due to regional hypoxia, regional hypocapnia, or to liberation of vasoactive substances such as serotonin and histamine. The latter are contained in and released from the platelets comprising the embolus. Local atelectasis and pulmonary edema may occur within 24 hours of embolization due to the loss of surfactant.

Clinical Manifestations

Pulmonary embolism produces three clinical syndromes, acute occlusion without infarction, acute pulmonary infarction, and acute massive occlusion. Clinical manifestations vary with the extent of the lung tissue involved. However, manifestations are often nonspecific and transient, so diagnosis may not be clear cut. Pulmonary embolism is frequently called the great imitator because the symptoms suggest other problems.

Signs and symptoms of acute occlusion without infarction include sudden onset of mild, moderate, or even severe transient dyspnea not proportional to physical findings; substernal chest pain of abrupt onset; cough; wheezing; tachypnea, which may be transient and accompanied by hypocarbia; tachycardia, and anxiety. Acute pulmonary infarction occurs in less than 10% of patients with pulmonary embolism. It is associated with fever of 101° to 103°, cough, hemoptysis, acute pleuritic chest pain, pleural effusion, and pleural friction rub. Manifestations of acute massive occlusion are systemic hypotension; shock; diaphoresis; decreased organ perfusion; oliguria; dyspnea; tachycardia, and tachypnea.

The diagnostic aids used for detecting deep vein thrombosis are integral in assessing a patient with suspected pulmonary emboli. Other tests include arterial blood gas analysis; laboratory tests; chest x-ray; ECG; radioisotope scanning, and pulmonary angiogram.

Although the most characteristic arterial blood gas abnormalities following pulmonary embolization are hypoxemia, hypocarbia, and acute respiratory alkalosis, a variety of arterial blood gas abnormalities are associated with pulmonary emboli. None of the abnormalities are sufficiently sensitive nor specific to confirm the diagnosis. This is because arterial blood gas values associated with pulmonary emboli depend upon the size and location of the emboli, the existence of preexisting cardiopulmonary disease, and the amount of time lapsed since embolization.

No laboratory tests are either sensitive or specific indicators of pulmonary embolism. However, some, such as a complete blood count, LDH, SGOT, and bilirubin, suggest the diagnosis and differentiate it from pneumonia and acute myocardial infarction. Similarly, chest x-ray and ECG can suggest the diagnosis.

Perfusion lung scan is a highly sensitive but nonspecific test, and a negative scan rules out the possibility of pulmonary embolism. A positive scan indicates the need for a ventilation lung scan for increased specificity.

While pulmonary angiography is currently the most definitive test for diagnosing pulmonary embolism, it is associated with a 4% complication rate and a mortality rate of 0.5%. Ultrasound may become the most reliable noninvasive test of the future.

Preventive Nursing Interventions

Pulmonary emboli originate in the lower extremities. Therefore, interventions that minimize and/or prevent pulmonary emboli are the same as those that prevent deep vein thrombosis.

Therapy

Further embolization is the greatest danger for patients who survive the first few hours. Therefore, treatment is aimed at minimizing further embolization, preventing dislodgement and cephalad migration of blood clots, and alleviating the symptoms associated with the embolism.

The patient is kept on bed rest with legs elevated 10 to 15 degrees. The length of time that the patient is on bed rest is controversial, but should be continued as long as the patient has any signs and symptoms of thrombophlebitis or pulmonary distress.

If a patient is hypotensive, crystalloids are given. Hypotension due to low cardiac output may require treatment with isoproterenol, dopamine, or dobutamine. Digitalis is ordered for cardiac failure.

Oxygen, administered at 4 to 10 liters per minute by nasal cannula, eases breathing and alleviates or minimizes the symptoms of hypoxemia in most patients. Additionally, the head of the bed is elevated 30 to 45 degrees to improve chest expansion and facilitate breathing. If the patient has chronic lung disease, oxygen therapy is begun with a 24% ventilation mask. Because a chronic low oxygen state maintains this patient's respiratory drive, a high concentration of oxygen may eliminate his respiratory drive, and he will stop breathing. Intubation may be necessary at times, especially if pulmonary edema develops.

Morphine sulfate is administered to alleviate severe chest pain and anxiety, provided there is cardiovascular stability. Equally important, the nurse calms and reassures the patient. Decreasing chest pain and anxiety may improve ventilation. Pain and anxiety can increase dyspnea, which in turn increases the patient's pain and anxiety. Bronchodilators may be needed if bronchoconstriction persists.

Cardiac dysrhythmias may also require treatment. The patient should be attached to a cardiac monitor.

Since most clots dissolve on their own, anticoagulation with heparin, the mainstay for treatment of pulmonary embolism, is given to prevent recurrent embolization. It may prevent extension of existing thrombi, but has no fibrinolytic activity and cannot lyse established thrombi. Heparin is given intravenously for 7 to 14 days following a loading dose. The goal of therapy is to keep the PTT values at 2 to 2.5 times normal. Patients with continued risk factors may be discharged on oral anticoagulants such as Coumadin for three to six months. For this therapy to be most effective, the Coumadin is started three to five days before the heparin is stopped.

Thrombolytic agents such as streptokinase and urokinase are used in instances of life-threatening pulmonary embolism, for example, a patient with massive pulmonary embolism who is in danger of dying and whose condition has not improved within hours of heparin therapy. A bacterial protein, streptokinase activates plasminogen, the precursor of plasmin, the naturally occurring fibrinolytic enzyme. Urokinase is an enzyme found in human urine and directly converts plasminogen to plasmin. Use of these agents for other patients with pulmonary embolism is controversial. Furthermore, use is contraindicated in patients who have had surgery or a biopsy within the past 10 days because of the increased risk of bleeding. Once activated, plasmin lyses not only the intravascular thrombus, but also the normal hemostatic clot in the wound. Initial thrombolytic therapy of 12 to 24 hours requires subsequent intravenous heparin therapy for 7 to 10 days.

Surgery is performed for one of two basic reasons: to prevent the migration of recurrent thrombi to the lungs, and to remove clots in the pulmonary vascular bed. Vena caval interruption prevents the migration of thrombi to the lung and is recommended for patients in whom anticoagulation therapy is contraindicated and for those who have recurrent pulmonary emboli despite adequate anticoagulation. Pulmonary artery embolectomy is indicated when a clot causes acute massive occlusion of 50% or more of the pulmonary circulation and when a patient is severely hypotensive and unresponsive to medical therapy. Figure 8-1 illustrates an approach to managing the patient with an acute pulmonary embolism.

Evaluation

The patient maintains adequate tissue perfusion.

| Fluid Imbalances

Postoperative patients are at risk for two extracellular fluid volume imbalances: extracellular fluid volume excess or extracellular fluid volume deficit. Extracellular fluid volume imbalances represent excesses or deficits of both water and electrolytes in nearly the same concentration as that of plasma. Despite changes in the extracellular fluid volume, percentages of water and electrolytes remain nearly the same.

Extracellular Fluid Volume Excess

A volume excess or hypervolemia occurs when the kidneys are unable to rid the body of unneeded water and electrolytes. Chronic cardiac failure, chronic renal failure, and the administration of excessive amounts of intravenous fluids, particularly those containing sodium, can cause hypervolemia in the postoperative patient. Whether caused by a dysfunction of homeostatic mechanisms or fluid overload, the result is the same.

Clinical Manifestations

Signs and symptoms of excellular fluid volume excess are myriad. They include puffy eyelids, peripheral edema, which may be pitting, elevated central or peripheral venous pressure, acute weight gain, and a full bounding pulse. Dyspnea and moist rales are late signs and symptoms.

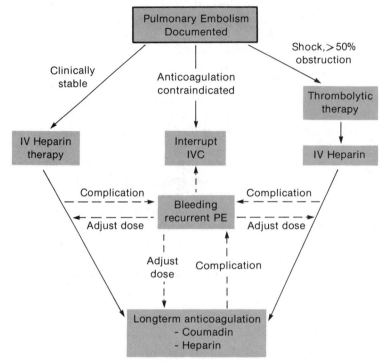

Figure 8-1. Schematic for the management of the patient with pulmonary embolism. (From Kinasewitz G: Management of thromboembolism. Chest 86(1):110, July 1984)

Preventive Nursing Interventions

1. Identify preoperative patients at risk, that is, those who have congestive heart failure or renal failure or who have received excessive amounts of intravenous fluids.
2. Monitor and record the patient's vital signs, noting increases in blood pressure and changes in pulse quality.
3. Monitor and record the patient's intake and output.
4. Administer fluids cautiously to patients with cardiopulmonary and renal disease.
5. Weigh the patient daily.

Therapy

Medical intervention for extracellular fluid volume excess is directed at eliminating the cause and alleviating the symptoms. Fluids are restricted, diuretics are administered, or fluids are restricted and diuretics are administered simultaneously. When the excess is due to the excessive administration of isotonic fluids, discontinuing the infusion may be sufficient therapy if the patient has functional homeostatic mechanisms. Strict intake and output records are maintained, and the patient is weighed daily and the results recorded.

Extracellular Fluid Volume Deficit

Causes of extracellular fluid volume deficit or hypovolemia in the postoperative patient include inadequate fluid replacement during surgery and excessive gastrointestinal fluid losses from nasogastric drainage, vomiting, diarrhea, and fistulous drainage. Systemic infection with fever and accompanying excessive diaphoresis and increased loss of water and electrolytes also cause hypovolemia.

Third spacing, in which fluid is lost from the intravascular compartment into the interstitial space or body cavities, causes an extracellular fluid volume deficit. Causes include handling the bowel or other tissue intraoperatively; decreased plasma protein levels as in liver disease with ascites; major abdominal surgery, and the increased capillary permeability that occurs in septic shock.

Initially in extracellular fluid volume deficit, water and electrolytes of the extracellular fluid replace the lost fluid and electrolytes. This reduces the extracellular fluid volume. Continued depletion of the extracellular fluid causes water and electrolytes to be drawn from the cells. Subsequently, a cellular fluid deficit eventually occurs.

Clinical Manifestations

Extracellular fluid volume deficit is often difficult to pinpoint because many of its signs and symptoms usually occur in a seriously ill patient. However, a most valuable indicator is longitudinal furrows or wrinkles in the tongue.

Characteristic signs and symptoms are tachycardia; increased respiratory rate; decreased venous pressure; orthostatic blood pressure changes, and thirst. Other signs and symptoms are dry skin and mucous membranes; poor skin turgor in the young and middle-aged patient; fatigue; urinary output less than 30 ml/hour with an increased specific gravity, and lack of moisture in the axilla and groin.

Weight loss can be especially helpful in diagnosing extracellular fluid volume deficits. A 2% weight loss indicates a mild deficit, a 5% weight loss, a moderate deficit, and a loss of 8% or more, a severe deficit. Additionally, in a severe deficit, hematocrit may be elevated because of hemoconcentration.

Preventive Nursing Interventions

1. Identify preoperative patients at risk, that is, those who have lost fluid and electrolytes in diarrhea, vomiting, or via gastrointestinal suction.
2. Monitor and record the patient's vital signs, noting increases in pulse and respiratory rates, and orthostatic blood pressure changes.
3. Monitor and record the patient's intake and output, including gastrointestinal, wound, and fistula drainage, and note excessive losses.

4. Be alert for longitudinal furrows in the tongue, poor skin turgor, and dry mucous membranes.
5. Weigh the patient daily, noting losses.
6. Administer fluids as ordered, assessing the patient frequently during the rapid administration of large volumes of fluid.

Therapy

Treatment involves providing both cellular and extracellular electrolytes and volume to replace losses without disrupting the composition of the extracellular fluid. An isotonic electrolyte solution such as Lactated Ringer's or isotonic saline is administered to treat a hypotensive patient with extracellular fluid volume deficit. Once the patient becomes normotensive, a hypotonic solution, such as half-strength saline, is ordered because it provides electrolytes and free water needed for renal excretion of metabolic wastes. Throughout the therapy the nurse monitors the patient for signs and symptoms of overload.

Evaluation

The patient remains normovolemic, experiencing neither an excess or deficit in extracellular fluid volume.

Electrolyte Imbalances

Hypokalemia

The balance of potassium, the major intracellular cation, is of primary concern because this electrolyte is needed for normal cardiac, skeletal, and smooth muscle function. A potassium deficit is common in the first 24 to 48 hours after surgery and reflects the body's response to surgical trauma with its physical and emotional stressors. This deficit is usually of minimal clinical significance and mirrors the mobilization of intracellular potassium and its excretion in the urine. After the second to fifth postoperative days, adrenal activity decreases. This results in a mild sodium and water diuresis and potassium retention.

Hypokalemia is associated with gastrointestinal suction, extensive bruising, wound healing, and the administration of potassium-free intravenous solutions to a patient receiving nothing by mouth. Surgeries, particularly those involving the digestive tract, cause the loss of potassium-rich fluid. Excessive diaphoresis and fever can also cause hypokalemia. Hypokalemia is often associated with metabolic alkalosis as potassium moves from the serum to the cells.

Clinical Manifestations

Because of its role in the normal function of muscle cells, the clinical manifestations of hypokalemia are those caused by muscle weakness. Early symptoms are nonspecific and include fatigue and malaise. A serum potassium of 2.5

mEq/liter produces such neuromuscular symptoms as weak, flabby skeletal muscles and decreased or absent reflexes. Cardiac dysrhythmias can occur, and prolonged hypokalemia affects intestinal muscle causing anorexia, vomiting, abdominal distention, and paralytic ileus.

Preventive Nursing Interventions

1. Identify preoperative patients at risk, that is, those taking potassium-losing diuretics, large doses of corticosteroids, and digitalis preparations; and those with fever and excessive diaphoresis.
2. Monitor the patient's serum potassium level.
3. Monitor and record the patient's vital signs, noting changes such as rapid, irregular pulse and hypotension.
4. Monitor and record the patient's intake and output, noting gastrointestinal fluid losses. Administration of even small amounts of potassium to patients with oliguria or renal insufficiency can cause hyperkalemia.
5. Observe a patient who is receiving digitalis for signs and symptoms of digitalis toxicity. Hypokalemia increases the sensitivity to digitalis and may precipitate digitalis toxicity.

Therapy

Depending upon the extent of the patient's potassium deficit, potassium may be ordered. Although the oral route is preferred, potassium may be administered intravenously.

Hyperkalemia

Hyperkalemia can occur postoperatively when excessive potassium is administered intraoperatively. Hyperkalemia is also associated with renal disease and may occur transiently in patients with normal renal function after major tissue trauma or after the rapid administration of stored banked blood. When red blood cells break down, they release their potassium into the surrounding fluid.

Clinical Manifestations

Clinical manifestations of hyperkalemia include vague muscular weakness and gastrointestinal hyperactivity including nausea, diarrhea, and intestinal colic. The serum potassium level is more than 5.6 mEq/liter. In severe hyperkalemia weakness and flaccid paralysis occur. A serum potassium of 7 mEq/liter causes bradycardia; a level of 9 mEq/liter, heart block.

Preventive Nursing Interventions

1. Identify preoperative patients at risk, those taking potassium-sparing diuretics, and those with infection.
2. Monitor the patient's serum potassium level.

3.   Monitor and record the patient's vital signs, noting bradycardia, or an irregular and rapid pulse.
4.   Monitor and record the patient's intake and output.

Therapy

The cause is treated first and the problem may resolve itself. All potassium supplements are stopped and the patient's serum potassium level is carefully monitored. Intravenous fluids are ordered because they dilute the potassium. Intravenous glucose, insulin, and calcium gluconate may be ordered to drive the potassium into the cells. Additionally, the administration of these medications may be followed by the administration of a potassium exchange resin. Sodium polystyrene sulfonate (Kayexalate) may be given orally, via nasogastric tube, or retention enema. Intravenous sodium bicarbonate may be ordered if the patient's blood gas values indicate metabolic acidosis. While being treated for hyperkalemia, the patient must be monitored for signs and symptoms of hypokalemia.

Hyponatremia

Hyponatremia in the postoperative period can be caused either by sodium loss or by water excess, which dilutes the serum sodium (water intoxication). In either situation, there is always proportionately more water than sodium.

In hyponatremia due to sodium loss, there is a sodium deficit, but no excess of total body water. Excessive sodium may be lost in gastrointestinal secretions via vomiting, diarrhea, or suction; in biliary drainage; in excessive sweating, or from the excessive use of diuretics such as thiazides or furosemide.

Because sodium loss lowers the osmolality of the extracellular fluid, fluid moves from the hypotonic extracellular fluid to the isotonic interstitial space. Thus the sodium in the interstitial fluid is diluted. As a consequence of the reduced sodium concentration in the extracellular fluid, potassium moves out of the intracellular fluid and the patient becomes hypokalemic.

Hyponatremia associated with water excess can be caused by inadequate excretion of water in relation to intake, and excessive intake of hypotonic solutions. Inadequate excretion of water occurs when extra antidiuretic hormone is secreted. Many factors inherent in the perioperative period cause the release of additional antidiuretic hormone. Such factors are pain, trauma, physical and emotional stress, and surgical stimulation.

Despite a low serum sodium, water is retained. Expansion of the extracellular fluid volume inhibits the increased secretion of aldosterone, which retains sodium. As a result, hyponatremia develops. Subsequently, the extracellular fluid volume expands and additional sodium is diluted. The usual symptoms of hyponatremia develop, and if the syndrome is not interrupted, cerebral edema results as osmosis draws water into the cerebrospinal fluid.

Excessive intake of hypotonic solutions can occur because of repeated tap water enemas; permitting the patient with gastric or intestinal suction to drink water freely; absorption of irrigating fluid during transurethral resection of the prostate, and parenteral administration of electrolyte-poor solutions. Because the osmolality of the serum is lowered, its water is pulled into the interstitial space and intracellular compartments and the cells swell.

Clinical Manifestations

Signs and symptoms of hyponatremia depend on its cause, severity, and rapidity of onset. Clinical manifestations of hyponatremia due to sodium loss include lethargy; anorexia; nausea; vomiting; headache; abdominal cramping, and confusion. Signs and symptoms of hyponatremia due to acute water excess are those listed, plus more serious neurologic signs such as convulsions and coma. Although the first indicator is depressed plasma sodium, signs and symptoms often appear after the patient is beyond help.

Preventive Nursing Interventions

1. Identify preoperative patients at risk, those receiving excessive intravenous fluids of dextrose and water, those losing gastrointestinal secretions, and those taking diuretics especially in combination with a low-salt diet.
2. Monitor the patient's serum sodium level.
3. Monitor and record the patient's intake and output, noting loss of gastrointestinal secretions.
5. Monitor the patient's urine specific gravity; it usually is very low in hyponatremia.
6. Monitor the administration rate of intravenous fluids.
7. Monitor the patient's neurological status for confusion.

Therapy

Treatment depends upon the underlying cause of the hyponatremia and the severity of the imbalance. When hyponatremia due to water excess is severe, water may be withheld and small amounts of hypertonic saline may be administered intravenously. Similarly, the underlying cause of hyponatremia due to sodium loss is treated, and fluids and electrolytes are replaced.

Hypocalcemia

Calcium is the most abundant electrolyte in the body. This cation is an important factor in coagulation, neuromuscular function, cardiac contraction, membrane integrity, and the electrophysiology of the excitable cells. Postoperative patients at risk for hypocalcemia are those losing calcium-rich intestinal secretions and pancreatic juice, those having undergone a parathyroidectomy or thyroidectomy, those with cancer, and those receiving multiple units of citrated blood. A serum calcium level of less than 4.5 mEq/L can result from the rapid administration of large amounts of citrated blood, because citrate combines with calcium, thus preventing its use.

Clinical Manifestations

Clinical manifestations of hypocalcemia include increased perioral and digital tingling; hyperactive reflexes; abdominal and skeletal muscle cramps, and positive Chvostek's and Trousseau's signs. Tetany and convulsions may occur. The plasma calcium is less than 4.5 mEq/liter or 10 mg/100 ml.

Preventive Nursing Interventions

1. Identify preoperative patients at risk, those with vitamin D deficiency, those with malabsorption syndrome, and those having a thyroidectomy or parathyroidectomy.
2. Monitor the patient's serum calcium and serum albumin levels.
3. Monitor and record the patient's vital signs, noting cardiac rate and rhythm.
4. Monitor and record the patient's intake and output, noting intestinal losses.

Therapy

Intraveous calcium gluconate or calcium chloride may be ordered. However, before administering these medications, determine the serum albumin level. Administering calcium gluconate or calcium chloride to a patient whose serum albumin level is low can cause hypercalcemia and cardiac dysrhythmias. If the serum albumin level is normal, administer the calcium preparation slowly to avoid causing cardiac dysrhythmias. Calcium is slowly infused with digitalized patients.

In severe cases of hypocalcemia vitamin D and phosphates may be ordered. Institute seizure precautions and evaluate the patient's neurologic status every 2 hours.

Evaluation

The patient's electrolyte values remain within normal limits.

Acid-Base Imbalances

Acid-base imbalances can occur in the postoperative patient for a variety of reasons. The cause determines not only the type of imbalance, but also appropriate preventive nursing interventions and medical and nursing therapies.

Respiratory Acidosis

This is one of the most common postoperative acid-base imbalances. The major factor predisposing the postoperative patient to respiratory acidosis is hypoventilation or the depression of alveolar ventilation.

A number of pre-, intra- and postoperative factors contribute to hypoventilation. Preoperative causes include depression of the central nervous system by drugs used to augment anesthesia, such as morphine, meperidine, or barbiturates. Intraoperatively, artificial ventilation may be inadequate to promote gas exchange. Postoperatively, the patient receives narcotics that depress the central nervous system, and he may not take deep breaths, sigh, or move, which predisposes him to atelectasis. Postoperative patients at high risk for respiratory acidosis are those recovering from abdominal or chest surgery and those with flank incisions.

Clinical Manifestations

Interference with pulmonary gas exchange leads to the retention of carbon dioxide, an increase in carbonic acid, and a decrease in pH. In uncompensated respiratory acidosis, the $Paco_2$ is elevated, the HCO_3^- is normal, and the pH is decreased.

Early clinical manifestations of acute respiratory acidosis result primarily from central nervous system depression. These include lethargy, weakness, drowsiness, and confusion. Additional signs and symptoms include nausea, vomiting, and headache. As the acidosis becomes more severe, level of consciousness may decrease.

Preventive Nursing Interventions

1. Identify patients at risk, those receiving CNS depressants, those with abdominal, thoracic or flank incisions, and those with pulmonary dysfunction.
2. Maintain a patent airway.
3. Monitor the patient's level of consciousness for lethargy and confusion.
4. Encourage the patient to deep breathe, sigh, turn, and ambulate, unless contraindicated.
5. Monitor and record the patient's vital signs, noting irregular pulse and respiratory rates.
6. Monitor arterial blood gas values (see Table 2-9).
7. Assess the patient's respiratory status before administering pain medication, and medicate the patient sufficiently so that he is able to move and cough.
8. Monitor the patient's intake and output so as to maintain an adequate hydrational status. This keeps respiratory secretions thin and clear, and easier for the patient to remove.

Therapy

Treatment focuses on maintaining a patent airway. Therefore, the nurse encourages the patient to deep breathe, sigh, yawn, and ambulate. Additionally, she suctions the patient as necessary and administers oxygen as ordered. She monitors the patient's fluid and electrolyte and arterial blood gas levels.

Respiratory Alkalosis

Respiratory alkalosis results from hyperventilation. This lowers the alveolar tension of carbon dioxide and disrupts the bicarbonate-carbonic acid ratio. Respiratory alkalosis is not infrequently encountered in patients being managed on ventilators and may also be encountered in postoperative patients who hyperventilate because of anxiety or pain. Other postoperative causes of alveolar hyperventilation include fever, shock, bacteremia, and pulmonary embolism.

Clinical Manifestations

The patient's pH is more than 7.45, $Paco_2$ is low, HCO_3^- is normal in the early stages, but decreases as the condition progresses. Other signs and symptoms of respiratory alkalosis include rapid shallow breathing, lightheadedness, dizziness, tingling in the fingers and nose, muscle weakness, and spasm. Because calcium does not ionize normally in an alkaline environment, the patient may have a positive Trousseau's signs or carpopedal spasm. Convulsions and came may also occur.

Preventive Nursing Interventions

1. Identify patients at risk, those who are anxious and those with fever, bacteremia, and in shock.
2. Monitor and record the patient's vital signs, noting rapid shallow breathing.
3. Monitor arterial blood gas values (see Table 2-9).
4. Medicate the patient for pain.
5. Identify potential causes of anxiety and work with the patient to minimize them.

Therapy

The treatment depends upon the underlying problem, but until the problem is resolved, protect the patient from injury. Keep the side rails raised and the bed in the lowest position. If the patient is anxious, calm and reassure him. Tell him to breathe slowly and explain why he should do so. Have him breathe with you. Start at his rate, but gradually breathe more slowly.

Metabolic Acidosis

In metabolic acidosis either the bicarbonate level decreases or the retention of hydrogen ions increases. Thus, metabolic acidosis is due either to a loss of bicarbonate from the extracellular fluid or to a gain of strong acid. Postoperatively the most common cause of metabolic acidosis is loss of intestinal secretions that are high in bicarbonate and sodium ions. Additionally, the formation of ketone bodies due to postoperative starvation, when the body uses its protein and fat stores as a source of energy, contributes to the gain of hydrogen ions. Other perioperative events that contribute to acidosis are shock; the rapid infusion of citrated whole blood; renal damage; hyperkalemia; severe infection, and fever.

The bicarbonate, pH, and $Paco_2$ levels are decreased. The buffers work together to buffer the excess H+ accumulated in the body. Occurring within minutes, hyperventilation causes a rapid decrease in the $Paco_2$ levels that may help bring the pH into a more normal range. When a rapidly increasing amount of metabolic acid overwhelms any respiratory compensation, the acidosis becomes more severe.

Clinical Manifestations

Signs and symptoms of metabolic acidosis are primarily related to its depression of the central nervous system. Clinical manifestations include weakness; vasodilation; deep, rapid respirations; stupor, and apathy. The patient's decreased level of consciousness may progress to coma.

Preventive Nursing Interventions

1. Identify preoperative patients at risk, those with uncontrolled diabetes mellitus, in a poor nutritional state, those losing intestinal secretions, and those with severe infection and fever.
2. Monitor and record the patient's intake and output, noting the loss of intestinal secretions.
3. Monitor and record the patient's vital signs, noting an increased respiratory rate.
4. Monitor arterial blood gas values (see Table 2-9).
5. Monitor the serum potassium level because it rises with acidosis.
6. Monitor and record the patient's level of consciousness.
7. Administer intravenous fluids and antipyretics as ordered.

Therapy

Treatment depends upon the basic underlying problem. However, protect a disoriented patient from injury. Raise the side rails, and put the bed in the lowest possible position.

Metabolic Alkalosis

This acid-base imbalance is due either to an increase in serum bicarbonate or a loss of acid from the plasma. In the postoperative patient, metabolic alkalosis may be caused by excessive vomiting, gastrointestinal suction, diuretic therapy, or hypokalemia. Loss of gastric juice results in loss of water, sodium, chloride, and potassium. Although the amount of sodium and chloride in the gastric juice will diminish if the vomiting continues, a similar loss of potassium in the gastric juice does not occur. Factors contributing to the extracellular alkalosis are continued potassium loss in the vomitus, the urine potassium loss in the early postoperative period, and a period of operative starvation.

Clinical Manifestations

The alkalosis increases the excitability of the central nervous system causing irritability, belligerence, and disorientation. If untreated, the alkalosis culminates in tetany and convulsions. As the body attempts to compensate, respirations become slow and shallow. The abnormal potassium level in the extracellular fluid may result in cardiac dysrhythmias. The pH and HCO_3^- levels are elevated.

Preventive Nursing Interventions

1. Identify preoperative patients at risk, those with excessive vomiting or gastrointestinal losses.
2. Monitor and record the patient's intake and output, noting the loss of gastric secretions.
3. Monitor and record the patient's vital signs, noting pulse rate and rhythm, and respiratory rate and depth.
4. Administer antiemetics to relieve nausea and vomiting.
5. Monitor arterial blood gas values (See Table 2-9).
6. Monitor the serum potassium level.
7. Monitor and record the patient's level of consciousness.
8. Irrigate a nasogastric tube with isotonic saline, not tap water. The latter enhances the movement of electrolytes from the plasma and interstitial compartments into the stomach from which they are suctioned before being absorbed. The result is electrolyte depletion or washout.

Therapy

Administer intravenous fluids as ordered, and if the patient has been vomiting, offer him isotonic fluids. Protect the confused patient from injury. Raise the side rails, and put the bed in the lowest possible position.

Evaluation

The patient's blood gas values remain within normal limits.

Genitourinary Complications

Urinary output during the first 24 hours after surgery is normally less than the 1200 ml to 1500 ml of urine that an adequately hydrated adult with normally functioning kidneys produces. The first voiding after surgery is usually about 200 ml, and surgical diuresis occurs on the second or third postoperative day.

For at least the first 24 to 48 hours after surgery the body retains fluid as part of its response to stressors inherent in the perioperative period. While increased catecholamine production results in an increase in the blood supply to the brain, heart, and skeletal muscles, it causes a decreased supply to the kidneys. Additionally, increased production of antidiuretic hormone and corticoids leads to retention of sodium and water, with a resulting increased intravascular volume. Similarly, increased aldosterone activity causes increased retention of sodium and water. These physiologic responses all contribute to decreased urine production.

Other factors also contribute to decreased urine production. These include the patient's preoperative hydration status, intraoperative events, and the effect of various perioperative medications. Preoperative dehydration, loss of body fluids during surgery, and an increased insensible fluid loss all contribute to decreased urine production.

Medications administered throughout the perioperative period affect renal blood flow and the production of antidiuretic hormone. General anesthetics cause a marked decrease in renal blood flow. There is a decrease in glomerular filtration rate and urine volume and an increase in osmolality. Other perioperative medications such as morphine sulfate, meperidine hydrochloride (Demerol), and Innovar decrease the glomerular filtration rate usually as a function of decreased renal blood flow secondary to decreased blood pressure. Regional anesthesia (spinal or epidural) causes minimal changes in glomerular filtration rate or renal blood flow as long as hypotension is prevented or treated with fluids.

While decreased urine production is normal the first 24 hours to 48 hours after surgery other events are not. Postoperative complications involving the genitourinary system include urinary retention and urinary tract infections.

Urinary Retention

Postoperative urinary retention is the inability to void spontaneously within 12 hours after surgery. This occurs even though the patient has normal kidney function, a full bladder, and no organic obstruction. Postoperative retention is usually transient and reversible.

Voiding can be initiated in two ways: triggering the stretch reflex and increasing intra-abdominal pressure. In detrusor voiding, bladder filling triggers the stretch reflex. Afferent impulses are transmitted and, if environmental conditions are appropriate, returning efferent impulses cause the detrusor muscle to contract.

Usually urine gradually collects until the bladder contains about 150 ml. The person then feels the desire to void. If he ignores this desire, he will feel the next sensation when the bladder is filled to the point of painful stimulation.

Physiological, emotional, and cultural factors play important roles in postoperative urinary retention. Perioperative medications such as narcotics and anesthetics dull central nervous system function and decrease the sensation of a full bladder. This, together with bladder atonicity caused by over distention, leads to retention. The use of epidural morphine sulfate for postoperative pain management is a highly significant factor in postoperative retention. The anticipation of pain upon voiding contributes to postoperative retention, especially when the operative site is near the bladder, urethra, vagina, or rectum. Positioning and nervous tension contribute to the inability to void as does lack of privacy, particularly if, in the patient's culture, urination occurs in private.

Factors predictive of patients at high risk for postoperative urinary retention are controversial. However, the following factors may be predictive: age; the surgical procedure; the route of anesthesia; alterations in fluid status; level of patient activity between the end of anesthesia and voiding time, and the amount of time that lapses between the end of anesthesia and the time of voiding.

Patients of advanced age are at increased risk for postoperative urinary retention. The older the patient the greater the risk of retention because of age-related factors (Chapter 2).

Postoperative urinary retention is also associated with the type of surgical procedure. For example, patients undergoing total hip replacement, intra-abdominal procedures, spinal surgery, vascular surgery, pelvic and perineal operations, hernia repair, lower extremity procedures, and hemorrhoidectomy are at increased risk.

The route of anesthesia also affects ease of postoperative voiding. Spinal anesthesia is associated with more postoperative voiding problems than other anesthetics.

Fluid imbalances have also been found to be predictive of postoperative voiding problems. Patients receiving minimal amounts of fluid can develop retention. The bladder fills so slowly that the detrusor muscle accommodates the increased volume in such a way that the stretch receptors are not completely activated. Conversely, the rapid administration of large quantities of fluids, particularly during the postoperative period, cause a large amount of urine to be stored in the bladder in a short time. During this time, central nervous system dysfunction can interfere with effective voiding and the bladder becomes distended.

The patient's level of activity between the time that anesthesia ends and the time that the patient voids is also predictive of voiding problems. The more active the patient, the fewer voiding problems he has. Similarly, the less time between the end of anesthesia and the time of voiding, the fewer voiding problems the patient has. In one study those patients who voided spontaneously did so within 2 hours to 10 hours after surgery.[3]

Clinical Manifestations

The major sign of urinary retention is the absence of voided urine. A distended bladder differentiates retention from oliguria or anuria. The distended bladder can be palpated above the level of the symphysis pubis. Percussion of a full bladder elicits a "kettle drum" sound. Conversely, percussion of an abdomen distended by intestinal gas produces a hollow sound.

The alert patient who has a distended bladder will complain of increasing discomfort and pain. He may be restless, anxious, diaphoretic, and hypertensive. (Normotension follows catheterization.)

The overdistended bladder may expel enough urine to relieve the pressure within it temporarily. The patient with a distended bladder who voids frequently in small amounts has retention with overflow.

Preventive Nursing Interventions

1. Identify patients at risk; consider age, type of surgery, route of anesthesia, and fluid status.

2. Avoid making the patient anxious as this may contribute to his inability to void.
3. Assist the patient to ambulate as soon as possible after surgery, unless contraindicated.
4. Turn the water on so that the patient can hear it. This may work via the power of suggestion and also obliterates the sound of urination. The latter may be very important to the patient if he has a roommate.
5. Pour warm water over the perineum or have the patient sit in a warm bath. These interventions may appeal to the power of suggestion as well as facilitate muscle relaxation.
6. Lightly stroke the inner aspect of the thigh or apply ice to the inner thigh. These actions may stimulate trigger points, thus initiating the micturition reflex.
7. Assist the patient to a normal voiding position, unless contraindicated. For example, help a male patient to stand and assist a female patient either to a bedpan placed on a chair next to the bed or to the bathroom.
8. If possible leave the patient alone when he urinates. Many people are unable to urinate in someone's presence.
9. If the patient can sit up or stand to void, having him lean forward or push on the abdomen with his arms or hands may facilitate voiding. These actions increase the intra-abdominal pressure.
10. Maintain a positive attitude, that is, that the patient *will* void. Do not threaten the patient with catheterization as the resulting increased anxiety does nothing to facilitate spontaneous voiding.

Therapy

Frequently the physician's postoperative orders will include "catheterize if the patient has not voided in 8 to 12 hours." However, catheterization should be performed only when other noninvasive nursing and medical interventions fail. Prior to catheterizing the patient, carefully assess the amount of fluid that the patient had during surgery, his preoperative hydrational status, and the time lapsed since surgery. Assess the patient's bladder for distention. Intermittent transurethral catheterization is superior to continuous drainage because of its lower associated infection rate.

Some doctors advocate percutaneous suprapubic bladder drainage rather than transurethral drainage for relief of postoperative urinary retention. The former has been used extensively in gynecological surgery and has a much lower infection rate than transurethral catheterization. Additionally, percutaneous suprapubic bladder drainage allows assessment of the patient's ability to pass urine spontaneously without removing the catheter. Other advantages are the elimination of urethral burning and discomfort and improved patient mobility. Disadvantages of suprapubic catheterization are mechanical complications and the fact that a physician must insert the catheter.

The physician may also order certain medications to help the patient void spontaneously. These may be administered either before a transurethral catheterization is inserted or after it is removed. Cholinergics and alpha-adrenergic blocking agents, if not contraindicated, may be ordered. Because cholinergic medications stimulate bladder contractions, bethanechol chloride (Urecholine) and Prostigmin may be ordered. However, they must never be ordered if the patient has a mechanical obstruction. These drugs increase intravesical pressure and could cause vesicoureteral reflux or a ruptured bladder, if the patient has an obstructed bladder outlet. If a patient is unresponsive to bethanechol, some physicians add an alpha-adrenergic blocking agent such as phenoxybenzamine hydrochloride to the regimen. This combination may result in effective voiding in patients with atonic bladders and functional outflow obstruction.

Evaluation

The patient voids spontaneously within 8 hours to 12 hours after surgery.

Urinary Tract Infection

The urinary tract is the most common site for nosocomial infections. These infections account for more than 40% of the total number of infections that acute care hospitals report. Nosocomial urinary tract infections affect approximately 600,000 patients per year. Sixty-six to eighty-six percent of these infections occur after manipulation of the urinary tract, primarily urinary catheterization. While not all catheter-associated urinary tract infections can be prevented, proper management of the indwelling catheter can prevent a large number of them.

Factors that determine whether a patient acquires a urinary tract infection depend upon the method and duration of catheterization, the quality of the catheter care, and the patient's health. Reported infection rates vary greatly. They range from 1% to 5% after one brief catheterization, to 100% for patients with indwelling urethral catheters that drain into an *open* system for more than 4 days. Although closed urinary drainage systems have drastically reduced the risk of acquiring a catheter-associated urinary tract infection, the risk remains substantial. More than 20% of patients who have indwelling catheters attached to a closed drainage system are likely to acquire infections on busy hospital wards. Host factors that seem to increase this risk are advanced age and debilitation.

Catheter-associated urinary tract infections are caused by both endogenous and exogenous microorganisms. Causative organisms include: *Escherichia coli, Klebsiella, Proteus,* enterococcus, *Pseudomonas, Enterobacter, Serratia,* and *Candida.* While many of these microorganisms are normally found in the patient's bowel, they can be acquired either by cross-contamination from other people, or by exposure to contaminated solutions and equipment. Regardless of their source, infecting microorganisms gain entry to the urinary tract via several routes. Catheterization can introduce those microorganisms inhabiting the meatus or distal urethra directly into the bladder. However, single, brief catheterization is associated with low infection rates. This may indicate that in healthy individuals, voiding or the antibacterial mechanisms of the bladder mucosa remove these microorganisms.

In patients with indwelling urethral catheters, microorganisms that cause urinary tract infection can migrate to the bladder along two routes. They can migrate along the outside of the catheter in the periurethral mucous sheath, and along the internal lumen of the catheter following contamination of the collection bag or catheter-drainage tube junction.

Clinical Manifestations

Clinical signs and symptoms of urinary tract infection include an elevated temperature and a foul odor to the urine. If the patient does not have an indwelling catheter, signs and symptoms are dysuria, frequency, and voiding in small amounts.

Preventive Nursing Interventions

1. Carefully select patients for catheterization. All of the estimated 4 million patients who are catheterized each year are at risk for catheter-associated urinary tract infections and its associated problems. Indications for catheterization include urinary tract obstruction, urinary retention, and the need to measure output accurately in critically ill patients.
2. Maintain a sterile, continuously closed drainage system. This is *the* most effective intervention for reducing the frequency of catheter-associated urinary tract infections. All other interventions are adjuncts.
3. Limit the handling and care of catheters to staff who aseptically insert and maintain them.
4. Insert catheters only when necessary and leave them in place only as long as needed.
5. Wash hands immediately before and after manipulating the catheter site or closed drainage system.
6. Use aseptic technique and sterile equipment when inserting a catheter.
7. Use gloves, drape, sponges, appropriate antiseptic solution for periurethral cleansing, and one-time use lubricant jelly packet for insertion.
8. Minimize urethral trauma by using the smallest catheter possible that ensures unobstructed drainage.
9. Secure the catheter properly to prevent movement and urethral irritation. If the catheter is to be in place only a short time, in either a male or female patient, or long term in a female, tape it to the inner thigh. However, if it is to be in place long term in a male patient, tape it laterally to the upper thigh or abdomen.

10. Disconnect the catheter and drainage tube ONLY if the catheter is to be irrigated.
11. Irrigate the catheter ONLY to prevent or to treat an obstruction.
12. Disinfect the catheter-tubing junction before disconnection.
13. Use a large volume sterile syringe and sterile irrigant only once; follow aseptic technique.
14. Obtain specimens of fresh urine from the aspiration port. Disinfect the port and aspirate the urine with a sterile needle and syringe.
15. Obtain larger urine volumes from the drainage bag.
16. Maintain unobstructed urinary flow. However, it is permissible to clamp the catheter for 10 minutes to obtain a fresh specimen.
17. Make sure the tubing is neither tangled nor kinked.
18. Do not allow urine to stand in the tubing.
19. Empty the collection bag at least every 8 hours, more frequently if needed.
20. Make sure each catheterized patient has his own collecting container.
21. Never allow the drainage spigot to touch the nonsterile collecting container.
22. Keep the collecting bag below the level of the patient's bladder at all times.
23. Never allow the collecting bag to touch the floor.
24. Change the catheter only when necessary, that is, if sandy particles are felt when the catheter is rolled between the fingers.
25. Daily meatal care remains controversial. In two recent studies, neither twice daily cleansing with povidone-iodine solution nor daily cleansing with soap and water were associated with decreased catheter-associated urinary tract infections.[4]

Treatment

Urinary tract infections are treated with the appropriate antibiotic. Other treatment measures include adequate hydration and proper bladder drainage.

Evaluation

The patient remains free of a nosocomial infection.

Gastrointestinal Complications

The postoperative patient is at risk for several gastrointestinal problems. These include acute parotitis; nausea and vomiting; paralytic ileus; abdominal distention; constipation; hiccoughs, and malnutrition.

Acute Parotitis

Acute parotitis, also called "surgical mumps," is a secondary staphylococcal infection that develops in the parotid glands due to extreme debilitation and poor oral hygiene. Postoperative parotitis accounts for one third of the cases of suppurative parotitis, and 90% of cases are unilateral.

Predisposing factors are: advanced age, that is, 65 years of age or older; malnutrition; dehydration; cancer, and avitaminosis. Onset usually occurs within 2 weeks after a major operation.

Acute parotitis results from a decrease in secretory activity of the gland. Parotid secretions become increasingly thick, and staphylococci, which are normally present in the distal third of the excretory duct of the parotid gland, migrate proximally. This process results in inflammation and an accumulation of cells that obstruct both large- and medium-sized ducts. Eventually multiple small abscesses form.

Clinical Manifestations

The first signs and symptoms of acute parotitis are pain, tenderness, swelling, and redness at the angle of the jaw. Progressive manifestations include a moderately high fever and leukocytosis.

Preventive Nursing Interventions

1. Identify patients at risk, those of advanced age, and those who are malnourished and/or dehydrated.
2. Provide good oral hygiene, that is, frequent gargles and mouth irrigation.
3. Ensure adequate fluid intake.
4. Stimulate salivary flow with chewing gum and hard candy.

Therapy

Treatment of early acute parotitis includes the application of warm moist packs, provision of good oral hygiene, and the administration of antibiotics as ordered. Severe parotitis may require incision and drainage of the parotid gland.

Evaluation

The patient remains free of acute parotitis.

Nausea and Vomiting

Nausea and vomiting commonly occur postoperatively. Causative factors include: preoperative medication; anesthetic agents; the type of surgery; obesity; electrolyte imbalances; gastric distention, and psychologic factors. Although postoperative patients are generally at risk for nausea and vomiting, some patients are at increased risk. For example, women between the ages of 26 and 56 are more likely to be nauseated and vomit postoperatively than are men, children, and the elderly. Obese patients vomit longer and more frequently postoperatively than do lean patients because fat deposits retain the anesthetic agents.

Vomiting is an involuntary reflex that enables the upper gastrointestinal tract to expel its contents via the esophagus and mouth when almost any part becomes overly irritated, distended, or excited. The stongest stimulus for vomiting is distention or irritation of the stomach or duodenum, but it can be caused by impulses arising in areas of the brain external to the vomiting center. Primarily a somatic nervous system function, vomiting is coordinated by the emetic or bilateral vomiting center of the medulla oblongata. Five mechanisms stimulate the emetic center. They are: the vagal visceral afferents; the sympathetic visceral afferents from the gastrointestinal tract, heart, kidneys, and uterus; the chemoreceptor trigger zone; the vestibulocerebellar afferents, and the cerebral cortex and limbic system.

The vagal visceral afferent pathways are stimulated by such events as gastrointestinal tract distention. Similarly, distention of the gastrointestinal tract stimulates the sympathetic visceral afferents from this hollow organ. This can occur postoperatively when fluid accumulates in the stomach, as when a nasogastric tube becomes clogged or the patient ingests food and fluids before peristalsis has returned.

Chemical substances, such as drugs, and rapidly changing body position stimulate the chemoreceptor trigger zone. Located bilaterally on the floor of the fourth ventricle, the chemoreceptor trigger zone informs the emetic center that noxious stimuli are present in the blood and cerebral spinal fluid. Rapidly changing body position stimulates the vestibulocerebellar afferents. The motion stimulates the receptors of the labyrinth of the inner ear and impulses are transmitted primarily by the vestibular nuclei into the cerebellum. From here the signals are sent to the chemoreceptor trigger zone and then to the emetic center.

The cerebral cortex and limbic system are stimulated by the senses, especially smell and taste, as well as by anxiety, pain, and various psychological factors. These stimuli cause vomiting by passing directly to the emetic center without involvement of the chemoreceptor trigger zone.

Once stimulation has occurred by one, several, or all these mechanisms, neurotransmitters conduct the stimulation to the emetic center. Stimulation of the emetic center results in stimulation of the fifth, seventh, ninth, tenth, and twelfth cranial nerves as well as stimulation of the spinal nerves to the diaphragm and abdominal muscles. The act of vomiting ensues. Initially the person takes a deep breath. The cricoesophageal sphincter opens, the glottis closes, and the soft palate lifts to close the posterior nares. The diaphragm contracts downward and the abdominal muscles contract simultaneously. The stomach is squeezed between the two sets of muscles and the intragastric pressure increases. Strong reverse peristalsis begins in the antral area of the stomach and moves the stomach contents toward the esophagus. Finally, relaxation of the gastroesophageal sphincter allows expulsion of the gastric contents.

Nausea is the conscious recognition of the subconscious stimulation of the emetic center or the chemoreceptor trigger zone. Nausea often heralds vomiting, but can occur after vomiting, or in its absence. Mediated primarily by the autonomic nervous system, nausea is accompanied by pallor; cold and clammy skin; increased salivation; tachycardia; gastric stasis, and diarrhea. There is also a somatic component to nausea. Swallowing movements often accompany nausea and are affected by the skeletal muscles.

Preventive Nursing Interventions

1. Move the postoperative patient slowly.
2. Encourage the patient to take deep breaths which facilitates removal of the anesthetic.
3. Keep the patient NPO until peristalsis returns.
4. Make sure that a nasogastric tube is patent and functioning.
5. Administer antiemetics, as ordered. Antiemetics such as the phenothiazines (Compazine and Thorazine) are believed to have an inhibitory effect on the chemoreceptor trigger zone. However, nonphenothiazines such as Emete-Con and Tigan are preferred by many physicians.
6. Provide pain medication, as needed.
7. Decrease fear and anxiety.
8. Monitor for electrolyte imbalances associated with nausea and vomiting, such as hyponatremia and hypokalemia.
9. Encourage the patient to use distraction, guided imagery, and relaxation exercises. These nonpharmacologic interventions are thought to inhibit or block stimulation of the cerebral cortex and limbic system. Additionally, when used with pharmacologic interventions the nonpharmacologic interventions can result in a reduced dosage of antiemetic, a reduction in the frequency of its administration, or a reduction in both dosage and frequency.

Therapy

Treatment of postoperative nausea and vomiting involves many of the preventive interventions. For example, the patient is kept NPO, antiemetics and pain medications are given, attempts are made to decrease fear and anxiety, and nonpharmacologic interventions are used.

Evaluation

The patient is free of nausea and vomiting.

Paralytic Ileus

Sluggish peristalsis, uncoordinated peristalsis, and even its absence, which is called paralytic or adynamic ileus, is not uncommon after surgery. They occur whenever the autonomic innervation of the gastrointestinal tract is disrupted and gastrointestinal motility is decreased. Causes include the stress response, irritation of the peritoneum, manipulation of intestinal organs during surgery, electrolyte imbalances, wound infection, and certain medications. In the perioperative period the physical and emotional trauma of surgery and general anesthetics trigger the body's stress response. Similarly, the handling of intestinal organs during surgery causes a sympathetic neurohormonal response throughout the entire intestinal wall that inhibits peristalsis. Electrolyte imbalances such as hypokalemia decrease gastrointestinal motility. And certain perioperative medications such as narcotics, that is, codeine, morphine, and hydromorphone (Dilaudid); anticholinergics, such as scopolamine, glycopyrrolate (Robinul), and atropine contribute to decreased peristalsis.

Sluggish peristalsis and paralytic ileus are temporary, usually lasting 24 to 72 hours. However, they can cause abdominal distention. Nonabsorbable gas accumulates in the intestine. It passes to and remains in the atonic portion of the bowel until the tone returns. When an unaffected portion of the bowel contracts in an attempt to move the gas, pain results.

Clinical Manifestations

In the first 48 to 72 hours after surgery, sluggish peristalsis or ileus causes slight abdominal distention, and bowel sounds are absent. Consequently, the patient passes neither flatus nor feces per rectum. The abdomen may become tense and distended. The patient may complain of fullness and diffuse pain and may vomit. Vomiting is not present in all cases of abdominal distention, but always accompanies gastric distention.

Gastric peristalsis returns within 24 to 48 hours after surgery. Colonic peristalsis returns after 48 hours. Peristalsis begins at the cecum and moves caudally. Mild cramps, the passage of flatus, and the return of bowel sounds and the patient's appetite, herald the return of peristalsis.

Preventive Nursing Interventions

1. Identify patients at risk, those who have had intestinal surgery, those who are hypokalemic, and those receiving narcotics and anticholinergics.
2. Assist the patient to walk as soon as possible after surgery, unless contraindicated. Walking hastens the return of peristalsis and minimizes abdominal distention.
3. Administer medications, as ordered.

Therapy

The patient is NPO until bowel sounds return. Medications such as dexpanthenol (Ilopan) may be ordered to increase intestinal motility and secretions.

A nasogastric tube or a long intestinal tube may be inserted to treat paralytic ileus that does not resolve within 48 hours. The tube must be patent and functioning properly and is usually irrigated with 20 ml to 30 ml of normal saline as needed. If a Salem sump is used, 10 ml of air are injected into the air vent (the blue pigtail) after the main suction lumen has been irrigated and the tube reconnected to suction. Additionally, accurate intake and output records must be maintained.

Normal saline, rather than tap water, is the irrigation fluid of choice. If large amounts of tap water are instilled, electrolytes move from the plasma to the interstitial fluid to the stomach. Once in the stomach, electrolytes are lost in the irrigant before being absorbed. Consequently, the patient suffers electrolyte washout.

Evaluation

Intestinal peristalsis returns within 48 hours and the patient experiences no untoward effects.

Constipation

Constipation results postoperatively due to colonic ileus from decreased gastrointestinal motility and impaired perception of rectal fullness. Constipation is primarily a problem of elderly postoperative patients, but may occur in any patient who receives opiate analgesics and anticholinergic drugs.

Clinical Manifestations

Early manifestations are anorexia and obstipation or diarrhea. The patient explains that he has not had a bowel movement in several days. His abdomen may be distended, and he may complain of feeling bloated and full. Other accompanying signs and symptoms are headache and nausea.

Preventive Nursing Interventions

1. Identify patients at risk, the elderly, and those receiving opiate analgesics and/or anticholinergics.
2. Keep the patient hydrated.
3. Assist the patient to walk as soon as possible and encourage frequent ambulation.
4. Increase roughage and fiber in the diet, if possible.
5. Administer stool softeners and cathartics, as ordered.
6. Monitor the frequency of the patient's bowel movements.
7. Provide privacy for the patient and ensure his dignity.

Therapy

Treatment of postoperative constipation involves the above preventive measures. Additionally, stool may have to be digitally removed and enemas given.

Evaluation

The patient's normal bowel habits return.

Hiccoughs

Hiccoughs (singultuses) result from intermittent involuntary contractions of the diaphragm, which is innervated by the phrenic nerve. These contractions cause an initial inspiration that is suddenly checked by closure of the glottis. The result is a short, sharp, inspiratory cough.

Hiccoughs are most likely to develop after abdominal surgery and are usually short-lived. Many factors contribute to their occurrence including those that irritate the phrenic nerve, for example, surgery near the diaphragm, peritonitis, and gastric and abdominal distention; anxiety; acidosis, and the presence of a nasogastric tube.

Clinical Manifestations

The classic sign of hiccoughs is the "hic" sound. Hiccoughs are generally more obnoxious than harmful. However, they can lead to exhaustion, vomiting, fluid and electrolyte imbalances, malnutrition, and wound dehiscence.

Preventive Nursing Interventions

1. Prevent abdominal distention by encouraging early ambulation and keeping a nasogastric tube patent and functioning.
2. Prevent acidosis.
3. Minimize the patient's anxiety.

Therapy

Treatment for hiccoughs varies from measures that increase the plasma carbon dioxide levels, to gastric lavage or suction, to the administration of tranquilizers such as chlorpromazine (Thorazine, Largactil). Gastric lavage or suction relieves gastric distention. If the patient's blood gas values are satisfactory, having him breathe in and out of a paper bag at 5 minute intervals increases plasma carbon dioxide levels. This increase depresses the transmission of nerve impulses that cause hiccoughs. Because tranquilizers have an antispasmodic effect on the diaphragm, they also may help relieve hiccoughs.

Evaluation

The patient is free of hiccoughs.

Malnutrition

In a temperate climate, a healthy individual needs 1500 calories daily to meet his nutritional needs. The stress of surgery and illness increases his caloric needs.

Postoperatively a patient who is being maintained on intravenous fluids of dextrose and water has only minimal caloric intake and no carbohydrate, fat, or protein. One liter of 5% dextrose and water contains between 180 and 200 calories.

The body responds to stress by increasing the production of glucocorticoids. These enhance the release of amino acids from muscle and mobilize fatty acids from fat stores. Thus, the patient loses weight as the body uses stored fat for energy. Ketonuria indicates that the body is burning fat. Similarly, unused amino acids are broken down into nitrogen end products and excreted as urea.

Unless contraindicated, the patient needs a postoperative diet high in carbohydrates, protein, calories, and vitamins. Nonprotein sources of calories are important. An increase in protein intake without an accompanying increase of calories causes protein to be burned for energy.

Preventive Nursing Interventions

1. Assess the patient's preoperative nutritional status (Chapter 2).
2. Identify patients at risk for postoperative malnutrition and prolonged negative nitrogen balance.
3. Ensure that the patient's preoperative nutritional status is adequate.

Therapy

Unless contraindicated, provide a diet that is high in carbohydrates, proteins, calories, and vitamins. Depending upon the patient's surgery, his preoperative nutritional status, and his ability to tolerate oral fluids and foods, the doctor may order total parenteral nutrition (Chapter 3) or dietary supplements such as Ensure.

Evaluation

The patient's nutritional status is adequate and his nitrogen balance is positive.

Integumentary Complications

Postoperative complications involving the integumentary system include not only wound infection, but also wound dehiscence and evisceration. Dehiscence and evisceration often result from infection.

Wound Healing

Wound healing is a fibroproliferative inflammatory process that repairs tissue defects. It begins at the time of surgery and continues for a year or more. The various phases of the cellular repair process are comprised of integrated and overlapping events. The listing on page 230 summarizes the phases, duration, and associated events of the wound healing process, and Figure 8-2 illustrates these events.

Tissues heal in one of three ways, either by primary, secondary, or tertiary intention. In primary intention, of which surgical wounds are an example, the incision is clean and straight, and all wound layers are approximated. These wounds typically heal quickly with minimal scarring.

In secondary intention, the wound edges cannot be approximated; granulation tissue fills in the wound. Wounds that heal by secondary intention have more scarring than do wounds that heal by primary intention. This is because more granulation tissue forms. Additionally, because wounds that heal by secondary intention (ulcers for example) are open, they are more likely to become infected.

The Phases and Events of Wound Healing

Stage	Duration	Events
I. Inflammatory (Also called the exudative or lag phase)	Day 1 to Day 3	Platelets adhere to damaged endothelial wall
		Fibrin deposited in wound
		Blood clot forms; hemostasis occurs
		Serum and white cells exude into area
		Wound becomes edematous; surrounding blood vessels become engorged
		Polymorphonuclear leukocytes and macrophages arrive
		Debris of damaged tissue and blood clot are phagocytized
II. Destructive	Day 1 to Day 6	Fibroblasts migrate into area and proliferate
		Polymorphs and macrophages clean wound
		Injured venules bud; new blood vessels grow
III. Fibroblastic (Also called the proliferative, connective tissue, or incremental phase)	Day 3 to Day 24	Collagen produced
		Granulation tissue forms
		Wound tensile strength increases
IV. Differentiation (Also called the maturation, remodeling, resorptive, or plateau phase)	Day 24 to Years	Vascularity of the scar decreases
		Fibroblasts shrink
		Collagen fibers enlarge
		Tensile strength increases
		Collagen in the scar increases and then gradually reduces

Adapted from Schumann D: The nature of wound healing. AORN J 35(6): 1068, May 1982

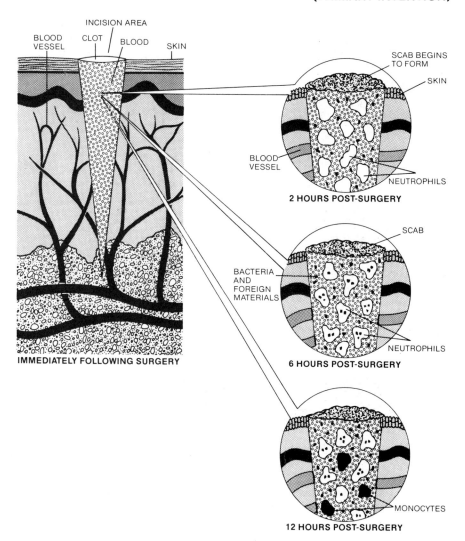

**HOUR-BY-HOUR VIEW
OF THE WOUND HEALING PROCESS
(PRIMARY INTENTION)**

Figure 8-2. Hour-by-hour view of the wound healing process—primary intention. (Courtesy Johnson & Johnson Products Inc.: Postoperative Wound Care, Part 1. New Brunswick, NJ, 1982)

In tertiary intention, a delay occurs between injury and suturing. The amount of granulation tissue that forms is more than develops with primary intention, but less than develops with secondary intention.

Wound healing is affected by a variety of internal and external factors. Internal factors include age; disease states; medications; nutritional status;

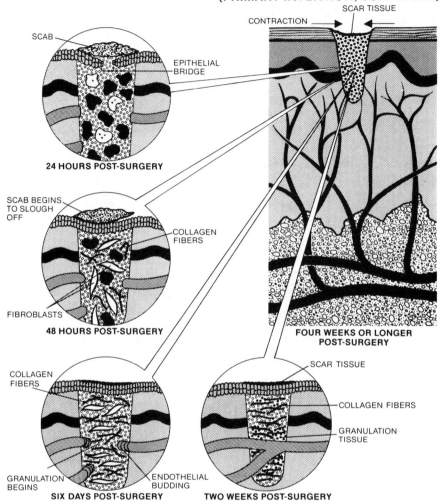

**HOUR-BY-HOUR VIEW
OF THE WOUND HEALING PROCESS
(PRIMARY INTENTION; CONTINUED)**

SCAR TISSUE

CONTRACTION

SCAB

EPITHELIAL BRIDGE

24 HOURS POST-SURGERY

FOUR WEEKS OR LONGER POST-SURGERY

SCAB BEGINS TO SLOUGH OFF

COLLAGEN FIBERS

FIBROBLASTS

48 HOURS POST-SURGERY

COLLAGEN FIBERS

SCAR TISSUE

COLLAGEN FIBERS

GRANULATION TISSUE

GRANULATION BEGINS

ENDOTHELIAL BUDDING

SIX DAYS POST-SURGERY

TWO WEEKS POST-SURGERY

oxygenation; stress, and vasculature. External factors affecting wound healing include the intraoperative environment; radiation, and drains and dressings.

Internal Factors

Healing takes longer in patients of advanced age. Fibroblastic activity and collagen synthesis decrease. Aging is also associated with other factors that delay healing, such as atherosclerosis, poor nutritional status, and decreased resistance to infection.

Diseases such as diabetes, with its circulatory and metabolic changes, delay wound healing. Similarly, chemotherapy delays wound healing, although the cancer itself may not interfere with healing. Liver disease adversely affects wound healing, due to decreased albumin production and decreased intestinal absorption of vitamin K.

Anti-inflammatory agents such as corticosteroids suppress inflammation, protein synthesis, wound contraction, and epithelialization. Prolonged use of antibiotics and cytotoxic agents retards wound healing, and aspirin decreases platelet aggregation and prolongs bleeding time.

Protein deficiency is associated with a decrease in such leukocytic functions as phagocytosis and immunogenesis. Vitamin A stimulates granulation of healing wounds, epithelialization in healing of skin incisions, and is essential for collagen synthesis. Vitamin B Complex acts as cofactors of enzyme systems, and vitamin C is needed for collagen synthesis, capillary formation, and resistance to infection. Vitamin K is necessary for the synthesis of prothrombin and various clotting factors, and zinc, copper, and iron all facilitate collagen synthesis. Obesity delays wound healing because fatty tissue has an insufficient nutrient blood supply. Additionally, adipose tissue is difficult to suture, thus increasing the potential for wound dehiscence. (See Chapters 2 and 3 for more information about nutrition and wound healing.)

Decreased oxygen to the tissues delays wound healing. Blood volume deficits lead to vasoconstriction and subsequent decreased oxygenation of the wound. Similarly, because smoking reduces the formulation of 2,3-diphosphoglycerate (2,3-DPG), it decreases the amount of oxygen unloaded at the tissues.

Prolonged physical and emotional stress are associated with elevated glucocorticoid levels. Cortisol inhibits wound repair. It alters the lymphocyte population, decreases eosinophils, basophils and monocytes, and degrades collagen.

Vasculature may be the most important internal factor affecting wound healing because an adequate blood supply is essential for wound healing. Any problems that diminish circulation contribute to delayed wound healing. The rate and quality of wound repair is proportionate to the local blood supply.

External Factors

An optimum operating room environment facilitates wound repair and recovery, thus minimizing wound infection. The latter delays wound healing because an infected wound will not heal.

Irradiated tissue is friable and subject to poor vasculature. Therefore, it does not heal well and is subject to infection. Additionally, heavy doses of radiation may cause wound necrosis.

Drains can facilitate wound healing by obliterating dead space and eliminating the accumulation of fluid. Drains are brought out through separate stab wounds rather than through the incision so as to avoid the development of fistulae.

Dressings can facilitate wound healing by optimizing epithelialization, reducing pain, and minimizing local inflammation and edema. Equally important, dressings enhance the physical and psychologic comfort of some patients.

Wound Infection

Surgical wound infection is the most common postoperative wound complication and is the second most frequent nosocomial infection in the majority of hospitals. Wound infections cause morbidity and mortality and may lead to other such problems as dehiscence, evisceration, fever, and septicemia.

Surgical wound infections are divided into two types, those confined to the incision, and those involving structures adjacent to the wound that were entered or exposed during surgery. Approximately 60% to 80% of infections are incisional. The remainder are at adjacent sites. This discussion is limited to incisional surgical wound infections.

A number of factors help determine the risk of infection. These include the degree of operative contamination, host factors, and local wound factors. Wounds can be categorized according to the likelihood and degree of wound contamination at the time of surgery. A widely accepted scheme categorizes wounds as clean, clean-contaminated, contaminated, and dirty or infected.

Clean wounds are uninfected. Inflammation is absent, and the respiratory, alimentary, genital, or uninfected urinary tracts are not entered. These wounds, which are primarily closed and may be drained with closed drainage, have a 1% to 5% risk of infection.

In clean-contaminated wounds, the respiratory, alimentary, genital, or urinary tract is entered under controlled conditions. Unusual contamination does not occur. The risk of infection for these wounds is 3% to 11%.

Contaminated wounds include open, fresh, and accidental wounds. Also included in this category are procedures involving major breaks in sterile technique or gross gastrointestinal tract spillage, and incisions, in which acute, nonpurulent inflammation is found. These wounds have a 10% to 17% risk of infection.

The category of dirty or infected wounds includes old traumatic wounds with retained devitalized tissue, as well as those in which a clinical infection or perforated viscera exists. They have more than a 27% risk of becoming infected.

Host factors that may lead to increased risk are numerous. They include age (either very young or elderly patients are at increased risk); presence of a perioperative infection; diabetes; severe malnutrition; obesity; the presence of devitalized tissue or foreign bodies; poor blood supply to the wound; protein deficiencies; vitamin C deficiency; a lengthy preoperative hospitalization; shaving of the skin the night before surgery, and a contaminated intraoperative environment.

Causative organisms include gram-negative bacteria and *Staphylococcus aureus*. Although 40% of the pathogens isolated from surgical wounds are gram-negative aerobic bacteria, *Staphylococcus aureus* is the species isolated most often.

Pathogens can be acquired from a variety of sources — the patient, the hospital environment, and personnel. However, the patient's own flora are implicated in most infections.

Exogenous contamination accounts for a large proportion of clean wound infections. Although personnel and the environment are potential sources of contamination, most infections result from the surgical team's direct contact with the wound.

Most infections are acquired from contamination in the operating room. If wounds are closed primarily and drains are not used, few infections are acquired after surgery. This is probably because most wounds seal within 24 hours after closure.

Whether a surgical wound infection develops depends primarily upon three factors

1. The number and type of organisms contaminating the wound
2. The condition of the wound at the end of surgery (surgical technique and disease processes encountered during surgery determine this.)
3. The patient's resistance.

Preventive measures are aimed at all three factors, but since most infections are acquired in the operating room, most preventive measures are aimed at influencing the surgical team. This is especially important since operative technique is the most important measure to prevent surgical wound infections. (See Chapters 3 and 6 for such preoperative control measures as hair removal and skin preparation.)

Surgical wounds do not usually become infected because of events occurring in the postoperative period. However, wounds can become contaminated and infected if touched postoperatively by contaminated hands or objects. Factors increasing this risk are an open wound and the presence of a drain. Until about 24 hours after surgery, when the wound edges are sealed, sterile dressings reduce the risk of such contamination.

Clinical Manifestations

Surgical wound infections usually occur between the fifth and tenth postoperative day, although they may appear as early as the first postoperative day. Specifically, wound infections caused by aerobic organisms develop about the fifth postoperative day, while those caused by anaerobic organisms develop between the sixth and eighth postoperative days.

Classic clinical manifestations of surgical wound infections are fever, increasing tenderness and deep pain at the wound site, and an elevated white blood cell count in conjunction with an erythematous wound. The wound rarely appears severely inflamed, but it is usually edematous and the skin sutures appear tight. Fatty tissue hides the presence of infection.

Infections caused by aerobic organisms produce a telltale temperature pattern. It spikes in the afternoon or evening and returns to normal by the next morning.

Preventive Nursing Measures

1.   Wash hands before and after taking care of a surgical wound.
2.   Do not touch an open or fresh wound directly unless wearing sterile gloves or using the no-touch technique. Once the wound is sealed, gloves are not needed to change a dressing.
3.   Remove or change dressings that are wet or if the patient has signs and symptoms that suggest infection.
4.   Make sure drains and closed wound suction devices function properly. Monitor the system regularly. Empty the reservoir at least every 8 hours. Maintain the security of the connections and note the color, amount, and odor of the drainage. During the first postoperative day the drainage will be sanguinous or bloody, but by the second day it will be serous. The greatest amount of drainage accumulates the first 24 hours and decreases until it ceases between the second and fourth postoperative days.
5.   Keep the area around the drain and tubing site clean.
6.   Keep drains and tubing away from the incision. The tubing can introduce infection into the wound.

Therapy

Treatment of infected surgical wounds involves the administration of antibiotics effective against the causative organism. A wound culture and sensitivity determine the antibiotic to be ordered. Additionally, the skin sutures may be removed and specific dressings and wound irrigations ordered. Half-strength hydrogen peroxide or povidone-iodine solutions may be used for irrigations. Both agents can inhibit bacterial growth in the wound.

Wet-to-dry dressings may also be ordered. A slightly moist gauze is applied directly to the wound. Dry layers of gauze without cotton filler cover the moist dressing. When this dressing is changed every 4 hour to 6 hours, the inner layer, which will have dried, is removed, bringing with it debris from the wound.

Evaluation

The patient's wound heals without development of infection.

Dehiscence and Evisceration

Wound dehiscence is the partial or total disruption of a surgical wound. A previously closed wound bursts, revealing yellow pink subcutaneous tissue. Complete dehiscence leads to evisceration, the abrupt protrusion of wound contents. Abdominal incisions are more likely to dehisce than thoracic incisions, with the exception of sternal wounds. Approximately 1% of abdominal incisions dehisce. Although evisceration most frequently occurs with abdominal organs, others may eviscerate.

Wound strength is stronger during the first three postoperative days than between the fifth and eighth postoperative days. The strength of the collagen framework is inadequate against forces imposed on the wound and dehiscence and evisceration are more likely to occur during this time.

Dehiscence usually results from a combination of both systemic and local factors. Systemic factors include advanced age; diabetes mellitus; uremia; immunosuppressive agents; jaundice; cancer, and obesity. Local risk factors include: inadequate wound closure; increased intra-abdominal pressure due to postoperative bowel obstruction, cirrhosis with ascites, severe coughing, and to chronic obstructive pulmonary disease (COPD) in which patients use abdominal muscles as accessory muscles of respiration; deficient wound healing, and wound infection.

Wound infection is a major factor in dehiscence. It is present in more than half of the wounds that dehisce. Additionally, a healing ridge is invariably absent in wounds that dehisce. A healing ridge is a palpable thickening that extends about 0.5 cm on each side of the incision. This ridge usually appears about a week after surgery and indicates that healing is adequate.

Clinical Manifestations

The discharge of serosanguineous fluid from a wound is usually the first sign of dehiscence. It occurs in about half the patients whose wounds dehisce, although occasionally, sudden evisceration is the first sign. The patient may also report a popping sensation after retching or coughing severely. The appearance of loops of bowel or other wound contents indicates evisceration.

Preventive Nursing Measures

1. Identify patients at risk, those who are obese and have abdominal incisions, those who have wound infections, and those who have decreased wound healing ability.
2. Minimize increased intra-abdominal pressure. Teach the patient to support the incision when coughing.
3. Keep nasogastric tubes patent and functioning.
4. Avoid wound infection.

Therapy

When a wound dehisces and/or eviscerates the nurse remains calm and stays with the patient. If an abdominal wound dehisces, she assists the patient to a low Fowler's position with knees bent to decrease abdominal tension. She checks the patient's vital signs and covers the extruding wound contents with warm normal saline soaks. She has another nurse notify the patient's physician. Although these interventions apply to both wound dehiscence and evisceration, urgency and risk of shock are greater with evisceration.

A dehisced wound that has not eviscerated is generally reclosed. However, the extent of the dehiscence and the patient's condition determine when it is closed. For example, if the skin is intact and the patient a poor operative risk, closure may be delayed indefinitely.

Evaluation

Surgical wounds heal by primary intention without infection, dehiscence, or evisceration.

| Physical and Emotional Discomfort

Postoperatively the patient is at risk for both physical and emotional discomfort. Pain and its control is a primary concern for postoperative patients. However, other discomforts to which the patient is at risk are confusion, alteration in body image, and fatigue.

Pain

Pain is a subjective experience that cannot be objectively measured. It has sensory, emotional, motivational, cultural, and cognitive components. Most importantly, it is whatever the patient says it is.

Pain has been categorized into two major types, acute and slow.[5] Each type has specific qualities and uses a separate pathway for transmitting pain signals to the central nervous system.

Acute pain is also called *fast pain, pricking pain,* and *sharp pain.* Associated with skin trauma, acute pain is not felt in most deeper body tissues.

Slow pain, or burning pain, aching pain, and throbbing pain, is associated with tissue damage. Characteristically difficult to locate and associated with autonomic disturbances, especially nausea, slow pain can occur both in the skin and in nearly all internal tissue and organs.

Pain receptors in the skin and other tissues are all free nerve endings. While superficial layers of the skin and certain internal tissues are abundantly supplied, most deep tissues are sparsely supplied.

Mechanical, thermal, and chemical stimuli excite pain receptors. Mechanosensitive pain receptors are pain fibers that are stimulated almost exclusively by excessive mechanical stress or mechanical tissue damage. Thermosensitive pain receptors are sensitive to temperature extremes. Chemosensitive pain receptors are sensitive to such chemical substances as potassium ions, prostaglandins, acetylcholine, histamine, serotonin, and the plasma kinins. Most pain receptors are sensitive to more than one type of stimuli.

Both acute and slow pain signals are transmitted in the peripheral nerves to the spinal cord, but at different rates. The pain fibers enter the spinal cord from the dorsal spinal route. They either ascend or descend in the tract of Lissauer and then terminate in neurons in the dorsal horn.

Two systems are available for processing the pain signals before transmitting them to the brain. One system processes the "fast" pain signals, the other, the "slow" pain signals. Despite processing differences in the spinal cord, both fast and slow signals pass to the brain via the lateral division of the anterolateral sensory pathway.

Approximately two thirds of all pain fibers end in the reticular formation of the brain stem. Higher order neurons are sent to such areas as the thalamus, hypothalamus, and cerebrum. However, some pain fibers, particularly those that transmit acute pain, go directly to the thalamus. Furthermore, although the slow pain fibers end almost entirely in the reticular formation, many signals are relayed to the thalamus. Because the slow fibers stimulate the reticular activating system, they affect the entire nervous system.

Pain impulses entering only the reticular formation, thalamus, and other lower centers are thought to cause conscious pain perception, while the cortex interprets its quality. Although the physiology of postoperative pain is the same for all patients, its perception or central integration differs. A key psychological factor affecting a patient's perception of pain, his tolerance and behavioral response is his experience with it.

Other factors thought to affect the pain experience are age, sex, and marital status. However, research results dealing with such factors are inconsistent.

Events of surgery, including incising, retracting, and suturing of tissues, cause cellular and tissue injury and death. Cellular and tissue injury causes the release of chemical substances into the surrounding area. Although normally barricaded from the sensory nerve network by cellular membrane barriers, when released, these endogenous substances stimulate pain receptors and evoke a pain response. These substances include potassium ions, prostaglandins, acetylcholine, histamine, serotonin, and the plasma kinins.

Other events that cause postoperative pain include tissue ischemia and muscle spasm. Ischemia, with its subsequent anaerobic metabolism, is thought to cause large amounts of lactic acid to accumulate, which stimulate the pain nerve endings. However, the pain may occur because the cell damage causes other chemical substances such as bradykinin to form.

Muscle spasm probably causes pain in part by directly stimulating mechanosensitive pain receptors. However, the ischemia caused by the spasm may cause the pain by stimulating chemosensitive pain receptors. Muscle spasm compresses the blood vessels, thus decreasing the blood supply to the muscle. Simultaneously, the spasm increases the metabolic rate of the muscle tissue, and the relative ischemia becomes even greater.

Acute postoperative pain is attributable to a definite cause and is self-limiting. Although the incision of muscle, fascia, and nerves causes the pain, several other factors influence its severity. Among them are the location and type of incision, the amount of retraction needed during the procedure, and the extent and duration of the procedure.

Incisions involving the upper abdomen and chest cause more pain because of the proximity of the diaphragm and lungs. Surgery involving the joints, back, and anorectal region causes significant postoperative pain due to muscle spasms. Furthermore, vertical or diagonal incisions cause more postoperative pain than transverse or S-shaped incisions.

The amount of retraction required to maintain exposure of the surgical site, and the length of time the retraction is needed affect the severity of postoperative pain. In terms of both extent and duration, less retraction is associated with less tissue trauma and less postoperative pain.

The duration and extent of a surgical procedure affects the incidence of postoperative pain. Prolonged procedures, even with the same incisions, cause more postoperative pain. Prolonged exposure causes trauma, stretching, and aeration of internal tissues, which in turn increase cellular lysis and injury.

Reflex inhibition, a disturbance in the gastrointestinal system, increases postoperative pain. Associated with extensive procedures involving tissue and organ manipulation, reflex inhibition results in abdominal distention, nausea, and vomiting.

Clinical Manifestations

Clinical manifestations of pain include such key physiologic signs as diaphoresis, increases in pulse and respiratory rates, and increases in blood pressure. Behavioral changes are restlessness and irritability.

Preventive Nursing Interventions

1. Each patient responds to pain in his own way. Therefore, postoperative pain relief begins with a preoperative pain assessment and preoperative teaching. (See Chapter 3)
2. Record the patient's baseline vital signs, as well as his activity level, affect, and body position.
3. To be most effective, pain medication should be given on a regular schedule, before the pain becomes severe. Furthermore, drug choice, dose, and interval between doses should be individualized. Effective use of analgesics not only relieves discomfort and pain, but also minimizes the development of such postoperative complications as atelectasis and hypoventilation.

   NOTE: Many nurses fear that patients will become addicted and therefore inadvertently undermedicate postoperative patients.[6,7] Patients are unlikely to become addicted. Studies indicate that most hospitalized patients stop taking narcotics when the pain is gone.[7] Therefore, patients should not suffer acute pain because medication is withheld to prevent addiction.[7]

Therapy

Treatment of postoperative pain involves the use of invasive and noninvasive techniques. The administration of medications is both the most common invasive technique and the most common technique used to minimize pain. Noninvasive techniques are electronic pain devices, comfort measures, distraction, and relaxation.

Invasive Techniques

Postoperative pain is a major concern for patients. Yet, inadequate pain relief and underprescription of narcotics are major problems for patients. The patient's comfort is the responsibility of the nurse. She assesses the patient and his pain and decides which interventions to use.

Before administering pain medications, the nurse assesses the patient's pain, considers the anesthetic used, determines when the patient was last medicated, verifies the medication administered, rechecks the patient's allergies, and checks his vital signs. The nurse evaluates and records the effectiveness of the interventions.

When assessing the patient's pain, the nurse
1. Considers the surgery that the patient had and how long ago he returned from the recovery room.
2. Asks the patient to describe the quality of the pain.
3. Asks the patient to describe the location of the pain. The patient may not have incisional pain, but rather pain from a full bladder, a too tight dressing, or from lying in one position too long.
4. Asks the patient to describe the intensity of the pain.
5. Asks the patient to describe any other sensations associated with the pain.

The nurse considers the anesthetic that the patient received, since it affects his postoperative comfort level. Inhalant-anesthetics, such as halothane, enflurane or isoflurane, with nitrous oxide and oxygen, offer little postoperative analgesia. A patient emerges from an inhalant-anesthetic within 5 to 20 minutes and usually needs a dose of parenteral narcotic in the postanesthesia recovery room. Conversely, balanced anesthesia, a tranquilizer, a narcotic, or both, plus nitrous oxide and oxygen, offers 30 to 60 minutes of postoperative analgesia.

The nurse must know not only the drug or combination of drugs that the patient received intraoperatively and immediately postoperatively, but also their effects and administration times. The tranquilizers used most often in balanced anesthesia are diazepam (Valium), lorazepam (Ativan), and droperidol (Inapsine, Droleptan). Although all produce sedation and potentiate the effects of narcotics, the duration of their effects vary. The effects of intravenous droperidol last 8 to 14 hours, while those of intravenous diazepam and lorazepam only 2 to 4 hours. Therefore, if the patient received droperidol, reduce the standard postoperative narcotic dose by one half to one third during the first 8 to 10 hours after surgery.

Although all the narcotics administered in balanced anesthesia provide analgesia and depress the respiratory system, the duration of their effects vary. The effects of intravenous meperidine (Demerol) and morphine last 2 to 3 hours. The effects of intravenous fentanyl (Sublimaze) last only 30 to 45 minutes. Therefore, if the patient received meperidine or morphine intraoperatively, he will probably need a postoperative narcotic analgesic 1 to 1½ hours after intraoperative administration.

The nurse considers the medication that the patient received previously, because narcotics can be subdivided into two groups, agonists and agonist-antagonists. An agonist, such as morphine sulfate, acts only as a narcotic. However, agonist-antagonists (Table 8-2) such as butorphanol (Stadol), nalbu-

Table 8-2
Narcotic Agonist-Antagonists

Drug	Dose	Equivalent to	Peak effect	Duration	Nursing implications
Butorphanol tartrate (Stadol)	2 mg IM	Morphine 10 mg IM	1 hr	3 – 4 hr	May precipitate a withdrawal reaction in patients physically dependent on narcotics
	2 mg IV		30 min	3 – 4 hr	
Nalbuphine HCI (Nubain)	10 mg IM	Morphine 10 mg IM	1 hr	4 – 5 hr	May precipitate a withdrawal reaction in patients physically dependent on narcotics
	10 mg IV		30 min	3 – 4 hr	
Pentazocine HCI (Talwin)	60 mg IM	Morphine 10 mg IM	1 hr	3 – 4 hr	May precipitate a withdrawal reaction in patients physically dependent on narcotics
	30 mg PO	ASA 600 mg	2 hrs	3 – 4 hr	
	180 mg PO	Morphine 10 mg IM			Use cautiously in patients with cardiac abnormalities

From Rogers A: What to expect from the most common analgesics. RN 46(5): 45 1983

phine (Nubain), and pentazocine (Talwin) can act both as narcotics and narcotic antagonists. If given to a patient who has been receiving narcotics even for only a few days, an agonist-antagonist can precipitate withdrawal symptoms and controls pain poorly. Yet, when given to a patient who has not been receiving narcotics, an agonist-antagonist produces pain relief.

Hydroxyzine (Vistaril, Atarax) and promethazine (Phenergan) may be ordered because they are believed to potentiate a narcotic or narcotic agonist-antagonist. Although given to increase either the effect or duration of an analgesic, most potentiators simply sedate the patient. Sedation is not equivalent to pain relief.[7,8]

Neither hydroxyzine nor promethazine potentiates narcotic analgesia. When given intramuscularly, hydroxyzine seems to have a potent analgesic effect, and when given with an analgesic, the effects are additive.[7]

Promethazine seems to have no analgesic effect, and when given alone, may increase the intensity of pain. When given with a narcotic, promethazine decreases pain relief. However, because promethazine causes sedation, it may appear to relieve pain. Discontinuing the promethazine and increasing the narcotic dose improves pain relief and decreases sedation.[7]

Nonnarcotics such as acetaminophen can be administered both with injectable and oral narcotics to provide effective pain relief. Narcotics act on the central nervous system. Nonnarcotics act primarily on the peripheral nervous system, although they exert some action on the central nervous system.

Although a common route of administration for analgesics, the intramuscular route is least advocated for pain relief. Intramuscular injections not only cause pain, but also may damage muscle and nerve tissue. Additionally, they are often poorly absorbed due to decreased muscle mass, lumps and sterile abscesses from previous injections, and varying injection techniques. Therefore, there is an increased use of intraspinal or epidural narcotics and of continuous narcotic infusion via a peripheral vein. Both techniques provide effective postoperative pain relief.

Intraspinal Narcotics.   When injected intraspinally, opiates seem to stimulate the opiate receptors in the spinal cord directly. The profound analgesia that occurs can last up to 24 hours and is not accompanied by anesthesia or sedation. Benefits of intraspinal narcotics include an improved quality of pain relief, decreased total narcotic requirement, improved respiratory function, and early ambulation.

Narcotics can be administered either by a single injection or by a continuous catheter. The narcotic is injected in the lumbar area at the L3, L4 interspace. Spinal cord injury is avoided at this level because the spinal cord ends at the L2 level. Additionally, injection at this level minimizes the rostral (toward the head) spread of the narcotic and the subsequent nausea and respiratory depression that can occur when the drug is injected into the thoracic or cervical areas.

Although the narcotic can be injected either into the subarachnoid or epidural space, it is more commonly injected into the epidural space. Injection into the cerebrospinal fluid-filled subarachnoid space is associated with respiratory depression, the leakage of cerebrospinal fluid, and spinal headache.

Side-effects associated with intraspinal narcotics include respiratory depression, severe pruritus, urinary retention, and nausea and vomiting. Although an uncommon occurrence, respiratory depression more often occurs with administration into the subarachnoid space than it does with administration into the epidural space. Due to the potential of respiratory depression, the nurse frequently monitors the patient's respiratory rate. The patient may be attached to an apnea monitor or may be cared for in an intensive care unit the first 12 hours after surgery.

Naloxone (Narcan), a narcotic antagonist, is kept at the patient's bedside. Repeated doses of naloxone may be needed to treat respiratory depression because the duration of intraspinal narcotics exceeds that of naloxone.

Antihistamines are used to treat pruritus. The etiology of urinary retention and of nausea and vomiting are unclear. However, nausea and vomiting are thought to be due to the spread of the narcotics to the emetic centers of the brain.

Continuous Narcotic Infusion.   Narcotics such as morphine, hydromorphone (Dilaudid), levorphanol (LevoDromoran), and methadone may be given via continuous infusion into a peripheral vein. They are administered with a volume control set and an infusion pump with an alarm.

The narcotic dose is individualized, and as long as the patient is alert and his respiratory rate is constant, the dose is adequate. Initially the narcotic dose is administered hourly to evaluate the patient's response. But as soon as the patient is comfortable, the narcotic is infused on a 4 hour schedule.

During initial administration, the nurse assesses the patient's comfort level and respiratory rate at least every 30 minutes. However, when the patient's comfort level and respiratory rate are stable, the nurse assesses the respiratory rate every 4 hours. The date, time, medication, patient's pain level, and respiratory rate are documented on a flow sheet.

Patients receiving narcotics via continuous infusion do not develop a psychological need as can happen with patients who depend on p.r.n. narcotics. Furthermore, the vast majority of postoperative patients stop taking narcotics when the pain subsides.

The switch from continuous intravenous infusion narcotics to oral narcotics is done gradually. An equianalgesic list (Table 8-3) is used. The nurse can facilitate switching a patient to oral narcotics. She makes sure that the oral dose of the medication is sufficiently large to relieve the patient's pain and that the oral dose contains the same amount of pain relief medication as the injectable dose. She gives the medication on a regularly scheduled basis, remembering that oral narcotics have a slower onset and a slower peak effect. When oral narcotics are given on a regular schedule, the dosage can be adjusted after a few days of around the clock administration. The dose can be decreased, and/or the time between doses can be lengthened.

It is important that the nurse tell the patient what to expect. That is, how, when, and why the change to the oral medications will take place.

Noninvasive Techniques

Electronic Pain Control.   Transcutaneous electrical nerve stimulation is used to provide postoperative pain relief. Two sterile electrodes are placed on either side of the suture line, parallel to it. A mild electrical current is transmitted to the nerves in the patient's skin. The mechanism by which electrical stimulation of the nerves produces analgesia is not clear. However, one theory suggests that the electrical current transmitted to the nerves stimulates the release of endorphins. They inhibit the transmission of noxious stimuli by attaching to opiate receptors on the excitatory neurons.

The electrodes are applied in the operating room, and the electrode wires are attached to the unit in the postanesthesia recovery room. When the patient awakens he adjusts the amount of stimulation, depending upon the amount of pain he is experiencing.

Side-effects with electronic pain control are minimal. However, they should not be used by patients with cardiac pacemakers. While the electronic pain control device may not affect the pacemaker, the pacemaker may interfere with the control device.

When using an electronic pain control device certain precautions must be observed. Do not place the electrodes over the carotid sinus because bradycardia can result. Additionally, avoid placing the electrodes over the laryngeal

Table 8-3
Narcotics

Drug	Dose	Equivalent to	Peak effect	Duration	Nursing implications
Codeine sulfate	30–60 mg PO	ASA 600 mg	2 hr	3–4 hr	Do not use intravenously
	200 mg PO	Morphine 10 mg IM			
Levorphanol tartrate (Levo-Dromoran)	4 mg PO	Morphine 10 mg IM	2 hr	4–5 hr	May cause oversedation, confusion, visual disturbances, and urinary retention
	2 mg IM	Morphine 10 mg IM	1 hr	4–5 hr	Contraindicated for patients with impaired pulmonary function, asthma, elevated intracranial pressure, or liver failure
	1 mg IV		15–30 min	3–4 hr	
Meperidine HCl (Demerol, Pethadol)	50 mg PO	ASA 600 mg	2 hr	3–4 hr	Causes CNS excitation ranging from irritability to seizures. Not for chronic administration in patients with renal dysfunction
	300 mg PO	Morphine 10 mg IM			
	75 mg IM	Morphine 10 mg IM	1 hr	2–4 hr	
	50 mg IV		5–15 min	2–3 hr	
Methadone HCl	20 mg PO	Morphine 10 mg IM	2 hr	4–5 hr	May cause oversedation, confusion, visual disturbances, and urinary retention
	10 mg IM	Morphine 10 mg IM	1 hr	4–5 hr	Contraindicated for patients with impaired pulmonary function, asthma, elevated intracranial pressure, or liver failure
	5 mg IV		15–30 min	3–4 hr	
Morphine sulfate	60 mg PO	Morphine 10 mg IM	2 hr	4–5 hr	May cause oversedation, confusion, visual disturbances, and urinary retention
	10 mg IM		1 hr	4–5 hr	Contraindicated for patients with impaired pulmonary function, asthma, elevated intracranial pressure, or liver failure
	5 mg IV		15–30 min	2–4 hr	

(continued)

Table 8-3 (Continued)
Narcotics

Drug	Dose	Equivalent to	Peak effect	Duration	Nursing implications
Oxycodone (with ASA: Percodan; with acetaminophen: Percocet)	5 mg PO 30 mg PO	ASA 600 mg Morphine 10 mg IM	1 hr	3–4 hr	Not available in IM or IV form
Oxymorphone HCl (Numorphan)	1 mg IM 0.5 mg IV 10 mg PR	Morphine 10 mg IM Morphine 10 mg IM	1 hr 15–30 min 2 hr	4–5 hr 3–4 hr 6 hr	Not available orally. Contraindicated for patients with impaired pulmonary function, asthma, elevated intracranial pressure, or liver failure
Propoxyphene HCl (Darvon, Dolene) Propoxyphene napsylate (Darvon N; with acetaminophen: Darvocet N)	65 mg PO 100 mg PO	ASA 600 mg ASA 600 mg	2 hr 2 hr	3–4 hr 3–4 hr	Overdose can be complicated by convulsions

From Rogers A: What to expect from the most common analgesics. RN 46(5): 46, 1983 or pharyngeal muscles, since this may trigger spasm and interfere with critical nerve function.

Although studies to determine the effectiveness of electronic pain control have yielded inconsistent results, the devices do reduce postoperative pain for some patients. Some patients need no analgesics, while others need minimial amounts. Being able to do something to control postoperative pain is thought to be a significant issue in determining the effectiveness of electronic pain control.

Comfort Measures. Simple comfort measures can help decrease the patient distress and anxiety. They may also decrease the medication required, while simultaneously keeping the patient comfortable.

Make sure the patient is positioned properly and is in good body alignment. Consider the position in which he was placed for surgery. If muscles were stretched or strained, position him so that muscle strain is not exacerbated and help him to change position at least every 2 hours. When he is lying on his side, place a pillow behind his back for support, a soft towel or small blanket between his knees to prevent pressure, and support his upper arm on a pillow. Furthermore, keep the sheets as wrinkle-free as possible.

Offer mouth care and ask the patient if he would like to wipe his face with a cool washcloth. Offer the patient a backrub, and if he accepts, position him comfortably.

Create a comfortable and restful environment. Adjust room light, temperature, and noise level to the patient's comfort level. Keep the patient's unit tidy and do not place the urinal or bedpan on the patient's over-bed table near his drinking water.

Spend time with the patient. Conversation, if the patient wishes to talk, can provide distraction and even if the patient does not wish to talk, the nurse's presence is reassuring.

Distraction. Distraction is a type of sensory shielding and is a potent pain relief method. Although the relief associated with distraction lasts only as long as the distraction, these techniques can be used effectively when the patient will have brief, sharp, intense pain, for example, during a dressing change or an injection. Depending upon the patient's likes, suggest active listening, conversation, rhythmic singing, rhythmic breathing, and guide the patient through the technique.

When the distraction ends, the patient will probably feel tired. He may also be more aware of the pain and ask for pain relief medication so that he can rest.

Relaxation. Relaxation, the freedom from mental and physical distress and tension, helps relieve fatigue, decreases anxiety, and relieves muscle tension. Additionally, relaxation techniques give the patient a sense of control over the pain and enhance the effects of analgesics.

A patient may practice relaxation regularly. If so, suggest that he continue to use his usual technique. If he does not practice relaxation, suggest that he try abdominal breathing or sighing and guide him through the technique.

Evaluation

The patient states that his pain is relieved, and he suffers no untoward effects from the techniques used.

Confusion

Postoperative confusion is not uncommon, particularly in patients more than 60 years of age. Confusion can not only frighten the patient, but can also threaten his physical well-being.

Postoperative confusion can be defined as an abrupt onset of disorientation, a disturbance in the awareness of time, place, or person. It excludes chronic or irreversible confusion and is transient and intermittent. A major physiologic or psychic imbalance is required for an acute confusional state to develop in a young adult. Conversely, only a minor shift is required for an acute confusional state to develop in an elderly patient.

Although its pathophysiology is not completely understood, confusion is a syndrome secondary to myriad causes. Some adversely affect the environment that supports brain processes. Although systemic in origin, the following affect brain cell metabolism: alterations in body temperature; decreased oxygen supply; malnutrition; accumulation of metabolites; fluid and electrolyte imbalances, and drug toxicity. Pharmaceuticals associated with acute confusion include tranquilizers; sedatives; digitalis; vasodilators; steroids; antihypertensives; diuretics; antidepressants; narcotics; antiarrhythmics, and bronchodilators.

The absence of meaning in one's environment also causes acute confusion. Lack of meaning can result from life-event changes, such as loss of a spouse or significant other, lack of social interaction or sensory deprivation, as well as sensory overload.

Other factors believed to contribute to confusion have been identified. They include a strange environment; altered sensory input; loss of control and independence; disruption of life pattern; immobilization; pain; disrupted pattern of elimination, and disruption of sleep patterns.

Clinical Manifestations

The patient suddenly becomes confused, disoriented, or delirious. Recent memory may be impaired, and he may be disoriented to person, place, and/or time. He may also be inattentive, dazed, stuporous, restless, agitated, or excited.

Preventive Nursing Interventions

1. Upon admission, identify patients at high risk for the acute confusional state. Factors found to be predictive of postoperative confusion are preoperative confusion present either before or

after admission; postoperative urinary problems; slow mobilization; pain, and/or the absence of clocks and television. Because myriad factors cause acute confusion in the elderly, initial assessment is imperative.

2. Throughout the patient's hospitalization reassess him for the presence of factors known to be associated with the development of acute confusion.

3. Maintain continuity in the environment and provide normal living cues.

4. Ensure that the same staff members care for the patient so as to maintain continuity for the patient.

5. Make sure the patient has clean eyeglasses and a functional hearing aid in place when needed.

6. Demonstrate a high degree of caring and concern for the patient. Use touch as appropriate. Provide privacy for the patient.

7. Encourage face-to-face interaction with the patient and call him by his preferred name.

8. Give the patient information about his environment and his plan of care. Help him have control over his environment and care to the extent possible.

9. Encourage ambulation and mobility.

10. Keep a clock and calendar in easy view of the patient.

11. Anticipate and prevent pain.

12. Assess usual elimination habits and patterns and involve the patient in planning to meet these needs.

Therapy

Each confused patient must be treated individually and symptomatically. Continue the nursing interventions listed above and reorient the disoriented patient frequently. Use medications and restraints only if necessary. Some medications increase the patient's confusion, and restraints can both alarm and agitate him. If the confusion is related to sensory overload, include time for rest and sleep in the patient's care plan.

Evaluation

The patient remains oriented to person, place, and time.

Alteration in Body Image

Body image is the mental picture that a person has of himself. Subject to both physical and psychological influences, body image is the foundation of a person's identity, self-esteem, and self-worth. It not only affects the way that a person thinks about himself, but also his relationships with others. A developed body image helps protect a person against life's changes and threats.

The development of body image is both a lifelong and interpersonal process. A person constantly differentiates, integrates, and expresses new experiences. He coordinates, unifies, and incorporates the sensory input of physical stimuli and of the socio-cultural environment.

Body image begins to develop in infancy and is modified throughout life. A person comes to distinguish between himself and the world and between himself and parts of himself.

In infancy a child builds a basic sense of trust. Through cuddling, holding, and feeding, the infant begins to form his identity and gradually learns that he is a separate being. A toddler learns self-esteem and positive self-regard. A child learns that he can do things for himself, and his parents and others stress learning gender identity.

Knowledge, trust, respect, and self-esteem continue to grow throughout childhood, and in school the child learns social interactions. Because his body grows rapidly, the child continuously adjusts to his body image.

Adolescence is a time of identity crisis. The adolescent is unsure of his wholeness and tests his boundaries. Peer pressure is strong and significantly influences an adolescent's body image. Gradually, however, the adolescent learns to cherish and guard his identity.

In adulthood, a person's body image continues to develop, but the need for reality testing decreases. An adult creates an environment in which he puts his trust and faith; he develops a relationship with a spouse or significant other.

Advanced age brings with it frequent reassessment of one's body image. Although a person has self-respect and dignity, he may be concerned about becoming lonely, dependent, and about dying. Additionally, as a person's physical condition changes and the possibility of physical crises increases, body image may become reduced or confused.

An interruption in a person's normal conceptualization of his body image leads to a disturbance in body image. A variety of physical, psychological, and emotional factors can lead to this disturbance. For example, illness, trauma, surgical removal of a body part, and medical-surgical treatments can cause an alteration in body image. The patient's perception of his body does not agree with his previously accepted body image, and he perceives this alteration in body image as a distortion of the self.

Many factors determine the extent of a disruption in body image and the patient's integration of this change. These factors include the patient's age, sex, personality, beliefs, expectations, values, and socio-cultural background. The most important of these factors, however, is the point in a person's life at which the alteration occurs. That is, what is the patient's age and stage of development, and what is the developmental task at this stage? For example, since a child is concerned with self-mastery and mobilization, disfigurement is not as threatening as a problem that interferes with goal attainment.

Other factors determining the extent of the disruption are the functional significance of the body part, its significance to the patient, the visibility of the body part, the amount of time that the patient has to prepare for the change, and his coping strategies and support systems, including relationships with members of the health care team. If the patient highly values the body part and/or it is highly visible, its loss can be quite disruptive. The amount of time that the patient has to prepare for the loss also affects the extent of the disruption. Lead time allows the patient to prepare for the resulting change in body image. This preparation reduces panic and excessive anxiety. Similarly, the patient's coping strategies and their effectiveness, as well as his support systems, affect the extent of the alteration in body image.

An alteration in body image, including its anticipation, triggers a series of natural emotional, perceptual, and psychosocial reactions. Alteration in body image arouses anxiety and emotional tension. These reactions may precede the change, occur simultaneously with the surgery resulting in the change, and occur after the change. The patient may feel insecure as his identity is threatened and his self-esteem is lowered. The alteration in body image can lead to depression and can combine with grief. Unless resolved, this combination can impair the patient's general physical and emotional health.

Threats to body image can disrupt not only the patient's usual life activities, but also may adversely affect his relationships with other people, including significant others. Additionally, an alteration in body image may change the patient's social responses and lead to stigmatization.

The mourning that can occur for a lost body part is similar to that which occurs when a person dies. If a patient undergoes disfiguring surgery, he is threatened by rejection and separation from significant others. However, these feelings dissipate as the patient reintegrates the changes into his total body image.

Preventive Nursing Interventions

The nurse must understand the challenge that an alteration in body image presents to a patient, for she is in a strategic position to promote the patient's recovery. Awareness of the patient's needs and sensitive planning and knowledgeable initiation of care can help the patient move from denial to acceptance and to integration of the change into his total body image. Preoperative preparation helps the patient and, ideally, a significant other prepare for the pending changes in body image and for both possible short- and long-term effects.

1. The nurse must be comfortable with her own body image, the meaning of certain body parts and of her feelings, and of the effect that she can have on the patient.
2. Identify preoperatively patients at risk for alterations in body image. Patients at highest risk are those who have minimal support and those who are dissatisfied with their body image preoperatively.
3. Assess the meaning of the alteration in body image to the patient. This is vitally important and must not be assumed. For example, a woman with ulcerative colitis may welcome an ileostomy because it will enable her to live a normal life.

Similarly, a woman having a hysterectomy may not be upset, and may not perceive it to be a threat to her femininity.

4. Identify the patient's coping strategies and support systems, and until learning differently, assume that the patient is coping.

5. The nurse caring for the patient should develop the care plan to ensure continuity and collaboration with other members of the health care team.

6. Provide the patient and family with sustained support and caring, and ask them if they would like to talk with a person who has successfully adapted to a similar alteration in body image.

7. Listen to the patient and encourage him to discuss his feelings, thoughts, and anxieties. Use open ended questions to facilitate this process.

8. Be attentive to the patient's behavior. If he is in the denial phase, accept it, but do not reinforce it. Reassure the patient that his reactions and feelings are normal.

9. Avoid arguing with the patient, and do not overload him with information.

10. Provide the patient with clear, honest, and direct answers to his questions.

11. Allow the patient as much control and decision-making power as possible. Depending upon his surgery, he may have lost some control over himself, time, or the physical environment.

12. Assure the patient that he can manage the situation successfully.

13. Assure him that he will be the same person after surgery that he was before surgery.

14. Ensure time and privacy for both the patient and his family.

15. Listen to the family, and observe their interactions with the patient. Encourage them to express their feelings, and help them talk with the patient.

Postoperatively, the nurse uses the same interventions as above. Additional interventions include:

1. Encourage the patient's independence and work with him to develop the most practical plan of care, which he may also use at home. This will enable him to regain feelings of self-worth and self-esteem.

2. Accentuate the patient's strengths, and minimize his limitations.

3. Help the patient anticipate the reactions and comments of others prior to discharge.

4. Tell the patient that he will still grieve for the lost body part when discharged. This is normal and the patient may need a year to complete the process. Help the patient identify support persons with whom he can talk at home, and also give the patient and significant other the name and telephone numbers of appropriate support groups and community agencies. If, after

one year, the patient has not integrated the alteration into his total body image and has not worked through the grief and grieving process, he needs psychiatric intervention.

Therapy

Usually the first indication that a patient is beginning to accept an alteration in body image is his looking at the area when the dressing is being changed. He then begins to ask questions about his care and to participate in it.

The patient then tests the reaction of other people to the change. By showing the altered part to others, the patient is asking them if they find the change as revolting as he perceives it to be. Supportive staff, family, and friends are imperative at this stage. For, by accepting the patient as he is, they facilitate his adjustment and make it easier for him to cope with the change and integrate it into his body image.

Despite pre- and postoperative interventions and the development of a therapeutic relationship, the use of appropriate communication techniques, patient education, collaboration with other members of the health care team, and provision of physical care, some patients may experience a crisis. Symptoms include extreme anxiety, depression, guilt, and/or denial of the situation. A patient's inability to accept reality may be the most significant block to recovery. It challenges all care-givers, and the patient needs counseling.

Evaluation

The patient successfully incorporates changes into his body image.

Fatigue

The postoperative fatigue syndrome is common even after routine operative procedures. In one study approximately two thirds of patients who underwent uncomplicated abdominal surgery complained of pronounced fatigue that persisted for at least 4 weeks after surgery.[9] In another study, one third of patients undergoing uncomplicated abdominal surgery experienced fatigue throughout the first postoperative month.[10] Yet other study results indicate progressive deterioration in psychomotor function during the first 4 to 5 days after elective surgery.[11] Although maximum on the fifth day, the deterioration persisted from 14 to more than 21 days.

Although the fatigue state has not been adequately defined and its pathogenesis remains unknown, postoperative fatigue has been found to correlate with such catabolic changes as weight loss, loss in triceps skinfold caliper and arm muscle circumference, and a decrease in serum transferrin concentration. However, the occurrence of postoperative fatigue has not been found to correlate with such pre- and intraoperative factors as age, sex, nutritional status, preoperative fatigue, and duration of surgery.

Postoperative weight loss is usually due to a combination of factors. Energy expenditure is increased postoperatively due to the body's physiologic response to stressors and a decreased dietary intake. However, findings suggest that factors other than the acute stress response or a subclinical postoperative complication cause the postoperative fatigue syndrome. Potential factors may include a combination of inactivity and the supine position. Additional research aimed at evaluating pathogenic factors and treatment of postoperative fatigue should focus on the mechanism leading to impaired postoperative nutritional status and muscle function.

Preventive Nursing Interventions

Specific preventive nursing interventions will be determined by further research. However, the nurse teaches the patient to pace himself and to increase his activity level gradually.

Therapy

Given that postoperative catabolic changes seem to be important in the development of postoperative fatigue, therapeutic measures should be focused on converting postoperative catabolism to anabolism. Although various techniques may attain this goal, enteral or parenteral nutrition seems most promising. Yet another suggested supplementary technique is regional (epidural) analgesia during and after surgery. Afferent neurogenic blockade inhibits the body's physiologic response to stressors of the perioperative period and improves nitrogen balance.

Evaluation

The patient experiences minimal fatigue.

Summary

Plans for achieving a complication-free recovery begin with preoperative patient assessment, the identification of factors that increase the patient's risk for surgery, and with proper physical and emotional preparation of the patient. It is in the postoperative phase that the nurse is able to evaluate the attainment of this goal. Outcome criteria for the patient in the postoperative phase are listed below.

**Outcome Criteria for a
Patient in the Postoperative Phase**

1. The patient coughs effectively and maintains a clear airway.
2. The patient resumes normal bowel habits.
3. The patient's breathing pattern is symmetrical.
4. The patient is free of postoperative pain.
5. The patient's fluid intake and output are balanced.
6. The patient's tissues are adequately perfused.

7. The surgical wound heals without infection.

8. The patient remains free of nosocomial infections.

9. The patient begins to adapt to alterations in body image.

10. The patient's nutritional status is adequate to meet body demands.

11. The patient achieves restful sleep.

12. The patient demonstrates the correct use of appliances, prostheses, and assistive devices needed to achieve self-care.

References

1. Haimovici H: Vascular Emergencies. New York, Appleton-Century-Crofts, 1982

2. Turpie AGG, Hirsh J: Venous thromboembolism: Current concepts — Part 2. Hosp Med 13–41, November 1984

3. Innes B, Bruya MA: Postoperative voiding patterns and related contributing factors. Washington State J Nurs Summer/Fall: 13–16, 1977

4. Wong ES: Guidelines for Prevention of Catheter-Associated Urinary Tract Infections. Atlanta, U.S. Department of Health and Human Services Public Health Service Centers for Disease Control, February 1981

5. Guyton AC: Textbook of Medical Physiology, 7th ed. Philadelphia, WB Saunders, 1986

6. Cohen FL: Postsurgical pain relief: Patients' status and nurses' medication choices. Pain 9(2): 265–274, October 1980

7. McCaffery M: Patients shouldn't have to suffer: How to relieve pain with injectable narcotics. Nurs 80 10(10): 34–39, 1980

8. Heidrich G, Perry S: Helping the patient in pain. Am J Nurs 82(12): 1828–1833, 1982

9. Christensen T, Bendix T, Kehlet H: Fatigue and cardiorespiratory function following abdominal surgery. Br J Surg 69(7): 417–419, July 1982

10. Christensen T, Hougard F, Kehlet H: Influence of pre- and intra- operative factors on the occurrence of postoperative fatigue. Br J Surg 72(1): 63–65, 1985

11. Edwards H, Rose EA, Schorow M, King TC: Postoperative deterioration in psychomotor function. JAMA 245(13): 1342–1343, April 3, 1981

Bibliography

Altered Image. Nurs Mirror 160(23): 46–47, June 5, 1985

Armstrong ME: Current concepts in pain. AORN J 32(3): 383–390, September 1980

Bailey CJ, Gulczynski B, Racky D, Vehrs K: Epidural morphine infusion. AORN J 39(6): 997–1005, May 1984

Baker AF: Clinical and laboratory management of pulmonary embolism. Geriatrics 38(4): 105–115, 1983

Barrett N: Ileal loop and body image. AORN J 36(4): 712–722, October 1982

Barrows JJ: Shock demands drugs — But which one's best for your patient? Nurs 82 12(2): 34–41, 1982

Baesl TJ, Buckley JJ: Preoperative assessment, preparation for operation, and routine postoperative care. Urol Clin North Am 10(1): 3–17, February 1983

Bender JM, Faubion JM: Total parenteral nutrition. AORN J 40(3): 354–365, September 1984

Besst JA, Wallace HL: Wound healing—Intraoperative factors. Nurs Clin North Am 14(4): 701–712, December 1979

Bobb J: What happens when your patient goes into shock? RN 47(3): 26–29, 1984

Brooks SL: Disturbances of bowel function. Nurs (Oxford): 871–876, 1984

Bruno P: The nature of wound healing. Nurs Clin North Am 14(4): 667–682, December 1979

Bullas JB: Fibrinolytic therapy—Nursing implications. Crit Care Nurse 1(7): 43–46, November/December 1981

Bullock BL: Restrictive alterations in pulmonary function. In Bullock BL, Rosendahl PP: Pathophysiology—Adaptations and Alterations in Function. Boston, Little, Brown & Co, 1984

Bullock BL, Ptak H: Fluid, electrolyte, and acid-base balance. In Bullock BL, Rosendahl PP: Pathophysiology—Adaptations and Alterations in Function. Boston, Little, Brown & Co, 1984

Cahill CA: Yawn maneuver to prevent atelectasis. AORN J 27(5): 1000–1004, April 1978

Campbell EB, Williams MA, Mlynarczyk SM: After the fall—Confusion. Am J Nurs 86(2): 151–154, 1986

Carey KW (ed): Caring for Surgical Patients. Springhouse, PA, Intermed Communications, 1982

Cerrato PL: Is your patient *really* ready for surgery? RN 48(6): 69–70, 1985

Chaudry IH, Clemens MG, Baue AE: Alterations in cell function with ischemia and shock and their correction. Arch Surg 116(10): 1309–1317, 1981

Chisholm SE, Deniston OL, Igrisan RM, Barbus AJ: Prevalence of confusion in elderly hospitalized patients. J Gerontol Nurs 8(2): 87–96, 1982

Christensen T, Bendix T, Kehlet H: Fatigue and cardiorespiratory function following abdominal surgery. Br J Surg 69(7): 417–419, 1982

Christensen T, Hougard F, Kehlet H: Influence of pre- and intra- operative factors on the occurrence of postoperative fatigue. Br J Surg 72(1): 63–65, 1985

Christensen T, Kehlet H: Postoperative fatigue and changes in nutritional status. Br J Surg 71(6): 473–476, 1984

Christensen T, Wulff C, Fuglsang–Frederiksen A, Kehlet H: Electrical activity and arm muscle force in postoperative fatigue. Acta Chir Scand 151(1): 1–5, 1985

Chvapil M, Koopmann CF: Age and other factors regulating wound healing. Otolaryngol Clin North Am 15(2): 259–270, May 1982

Cohen FL: Postsurgical pain relief: Patients' status and nurses' medication choices. Pain 9(2): 265–274, October 1980

Cohen S, Wells S: Nursing care of patients in shock—Part 1: Pharmacotherapy. Am J Nurs 82(6): 943–964, 1982

Cohen S, Wells S: Nursing care of patients in shock—Part 2: Fluids, oxygen, and the intra-aortic balloon pump. Am J Nurs 82(9): 1401–1422, 1982

Cohen S, Wells S: Nursing care of patients in shock—Part 3: Evaluating the patient. Am J Nurs 82(11): 1723–1746, 1982

Cooke DH: Focusing in on pulmonary embolism. Emerg Med: 86–115, May 15, 1985

Cooper DM, Schumann D: Postsurgical nursing intervention as an adjunct to wound healing. Nurs Clin North Am 14(4): 713–726, December 1979

Covelli HD, Weled BJ, Beekman JF: Efficacy of continuous positive airway pressure administered by face mask. Chest 81(2): 147–150, 1981

Cross M: Dissolving the threat of pulmonary embolism. RN 47(8): 34–39, 1984

Dantzker DR, Bower JS: Alterations in gas exchange following pulmonary thrombo-embolism. Chest 81(4): 495–501, 1982

David–Kasdan JA: An alteration in body image in the hemodialysis population. J Nephrol Nurs 1(1): 25–28, July/August 1984

DiNobile C: Wound drainage — Past, present, future. Today's OR Nurse 6(11): 20–26, November 1984

Drain CB: Managing postoperative pain . . . It's a matter of sighs. Nurs 84 14(8): 52–55, 1984

Ducey D: The phases of wound healing and wound irrigation. Point of View 20(4): 4–7, October 1983

Duroux P, Simonneau G, Petitpretz P, Herve PH: Therapeutic approach to acute pulmonary embolism. Intens Care Med 10(2): 99–102, 1984

Edwards H, Rose EA, King TC: Postoperative deterioration in muscular function. Arch Surg 117(7): 899–901, 1982

Edwards H, Rose EA, Schorow M, King TC: Postoperative deterioration in psychomotor function. JAMA 245(13): 1342–1343, April 3, 1981

Ellis BL: Predicting postoperative pain behaviors. Milit Med 143(12): 858–862, 1978

Eskridge RA: Septic shock. Crit Care Quarterly 2(4): 55–75, March 1980

Eskridge RA: The management of septic shock. Drug Intell Clin Pharm 17(2): 92–99, 1983

Fahey VA: An in-depth look at deep vein thrombosis. Nurs 84 14(3): 34–41, 1984

Falotico JB: Pulmonary embolism. Crit Care Update 8(1): 5–15, 1981

Fernsebner B, Baum PL, Bartlett C: Surgical prevention of pulmonary emboli. AORN J 39(1): 56–64, 1984

Flynn ME, Rovee DT: Promoting wound healing. Am J Nurs 82(10): 1544–1558, 1982

Folk-Lighty M: Solving the puzzles of patients' fluid imbalance. Nurs 84 14(2): 34–41, 1984

Foreman MD: Acute confusional states in the elderly: An algorithm. Dimens Crit Care Nurs 3(4): 207–215, July/August 1984

Frogge MH: Promoting wound healing in the irradiated patient. AORN J 35(6): 1088–1093, May 1982

Garner JS: Guideline for Prevention of Surgical Wound Infections. Atlanta, U.S. Department of Health and Human Services, Public Health Service, Centers for Disease Control, 1985

Gilmore IJ: Perioperative respiratory care. Urol Clin North Am 10(1): 65–76, February 1983

Glass LB, Jenkins CA: The ups and downs of serum pH. Nurs 83 13(9): 34–41, 1983

Glenski JA, Warner MA, Dawson B, Kaufman B: Postoperative use of epidurally administered morphine in children and adolescents. Mayo Clin Proc 59(8): 530–533, 1984

Gloeckner MR: Perceptions of sexual attractiveness following ostomy surgery. Res Nurs Health 7(2): 87–92, June 1984

Groszek DM: Promoting wound healing in the obese patient. AORN J 35(6): 1132–1138, May 1982

Guyton AC: Textbook of Medical Physiology, 7th ed. Philadelphia, WB Saunders, 1986

Hamer SS, Lemberg L: A complication commonly overlooked. Heart Lung 11(6): 588–592, November/December 1982

Heidrich G, Samuel P: Helping the patient in pain. Am J Nurs 82(12): 1828–1833, 1982

Henderson ML: Altered presentations. Am J Nurs 85(10): 1104–1106, 1985

Hockberger RS, Rothstein RJ: Pulmonary embolism. Top Emerg Med 2(1): 49–65, April 1980

Hoffmann J: Postoperative urinary retention. Br J Surg 71(12): 1007, 1984

Horowitz BF, Fitzpatrick JJ, Glaherty GG: Relaxation techniques for pain relief after open heart surgery. Dimens Crit Care Nurs 3(6): 364–371, November/December 1982

Huey R: 'Come quick! something's wrong with my husband.' Nurs Life 4(1): 33–40, 1984

Huffman MH: Acute care of the patient with a pulmonary embolism due to venous thromboemboli. Crit Care Nurse 3(2): 70–73, April 1983

Hunt TK, Jawetz E: Inflammation, infection, and antibiotics. In Way LW (ed): Current Surgical Diagnosis and Treatment, 6th ed. Los Altos, CA, Lange Medical Publications, 1983

Innes B, Bruya MA: Postoperative voiding patterns and related contributing factors. Washington State J Nurs Summer/Fall: 13–16, 1977

Jayne HA: Aspiration pneumonia. Top Emerg Med 2(2): 45–52, July 1980

Jung R, Wight J, Nusser R, Rosoff L: Comparison of three methods of respiratory care following upper abdominal surgery. Chest 78(1): 31–35, July 1980

Kalick SM: Clinician, social scientist, and body image. Clin Plast Surg 9(3): 379–385, July 1982

Keithley JK: Wound healing in malnourished patients. AORN J 35(6): 1094–1099, May 1982

Kinasewitz GT, George RB: Management of thromboembolism. Chest 86(1): 106–111, July 1984

Kotta CJ: Wound healing in the immunosuppressed host. AORN J 35(6): 1142–1148, May 1982

Lamb LS: Think you know septic shock? Nurs 82 12(1): 34–43, 1982

Lederer DH, Van de Water JM, Indech RB: Which deep breathing device should the postoperative patient use? Chest 77(5): 610–613, 1980

Locsin RGRAC: The effect of music on the pain of selected post-operative patients. J Adv Nurs 6(1): 19–25, 1981

Marta MR: Intraoperative hypothermia. AORN J 42(2): 240–242, August 1985

McCaffery M: How to relieve your patients' pain fast and effectively . . . with oral analgesics. Nurs 80 10(11): 58–60, 1980

McCaffery M: Patients shouldn't have to suffer: How to relieve pain with injectable narcotics. Nurs 80 10(10): 34–39, 1980

McCaffery M: Relieving pain with noninvasive techniques. Nurs 80 10(12): 47–54, 1980

McCaffery M: Understanding your patient's pain. Nurs 80 10(9): 26–31, 1980

McConnell EA: Clinical Considerations in the Use of the Vac-U-Care Closed Wound Suction Systems. St. Louis, Sherwood Medical, 1983

McConnell EA: Toward complication free recoveries for your surgical patients — Part I. RN 43(6): 31+, 1980

McConnell EA: Toward complication free recoveries for your surgical patients — Part II. RN 43(7): 34+, 1980

McConnell EA, Zimmerman MF: Care of Patients with Urologic Problems. Philadelphia, JB Lippincott, 1983

McCormack A, Itkin J, Cloud C: Preventing electrolyte imbalances. RN 32–33, November 1984

McGuire L, Wright A: Continuous narcotic infusion: It's not just for cancer patients. Nurs 84 14(12): 50–55, 1984

Metheny N: Preoperative fluid balance assessment. AORN J 33(1): 51–56, 1981

Metheny NM: Quick Reference to Fluid Balance. Philadelphia, JB Lippincott, 1984

Metheny NM, Snively Jr WD: Nurses' Handbook of Fluid Balance, 4th ed. Philadelphia, JB Lippincott, 1983

Morgan J, Wells N, Robertson E: Effects of preoperative teaching on postoperative pain: A replication and expansion. Int J Nurs Stud 22(3): 267–280, 1985

Moser KM: Thromboembolic disease in the patient undergoing urologic surgery. Urol Clin North Am 10(1): 101–108, February 1983

Moss JP: Historical and current perspectives on surgical drainage. Surg Gynecol Obstet 152(4): 517–527, 1981

Nicholson DP: Glucocorticoids in the treatment of shock and the adult respiratory distress syndrome. Clin Chest Med 3(1): 121–132, 1982

O'Brien J: Mirror, mirror, why me? Nurs Mirror 150(17): 36–37, April 24, 1980

O'Byrne C: Clinical detection and management of postoperative wound sepsis. Nurs Clin North Am 14(4): 727–742, December 1979

O'Donohue WJ: Chest editorials — Prevention and treatment of postoperative atelectasis: Can it and will it be adequately studied. Chest 87(1): 1–2, 1985

O'Donohue WJ: Special reports — National survey of the usage of lung expansion modalities for the prevention and treatment of postoperative atelectasis following abdominal and thoracic surgery. Chest 87(1): 76–80, 1985

Oakley L: Alterations in systemic circulation. In Bullock BL, Rosendahl PP: Pathophysiology — Adaptations and Alterations in Function. Boston, Little, Brown & Co, 1982

Ochsner MG: Acute urinary retention. Compr Ther 9(8): 61–67, 1983

Ochsner MG: Acute urinary retention — Causes and treatment. Postgrad Med 71(2): 221–226, 1982

Patras AZ: The operation's over, but the danger's not. Nurs 82 12(9): 50–5, 1982

Pearson, J, Dudley HAF: Bodily perceptions in surgical patients. Br Med J 284: 1545–1546, May 22, 1982

Pellegrini CA: Postoperative complications. In Way LW (ed): Current Surgical Diagnosis and Treatment, 6th ed. Los Altos, CA, Lange Medical Publications, 1983

Petlin A, Carolan JM: Before a runaway reaction — Halt hypovolemic shock. RN 45(5): 36–42, 1982

Podjasek JH: Which postop patient faces the greatest respiratory risk? RN 48(9): 45–56, 1985

Postoperative fatigue. Lancet 1(8107): 84–85, 1979

Rice V: Shock, a clinical syndrome—Part I: Definition, etiology, and pathophysiology. Crit Care Nurse 1(3): 44–50, March/April 1981

Rice V: Shock, a clinical syndrome—Part II: The stages of shock. Crit Care Nurse 1(4): 4–14, May/June 1981

Rice V: Shock, a clinical syndrome—Part III: The nursing care: Prevention and patient assessment. Crit Care Nurs 1(5): 36–47, July/August 1981

Rice V: Shock, a clinical syndrome—Part IV: Nursing intervention. Crit Care Nurse 1(6): 34–43, September/October 1981

Rice V: The clinical continuum of septic shock. Crit Care Nurse 4(5): 86–109, September/October 1984

Rogers AG: What to expect from the most common analgesics. RN 46(5): 44–46, 1983

Rose EA, King TC: Understanding postoperative fatigue. Surg Gynecol Obstet 147(1): 97–102, July 1978

Rosenow III EC, Osmundson PJ, Brown ML: Pulmonary embolism. Mayo Clin Proc 56(3): 161–178, 1981

Ross AD, Angaran DM: Colloids vs. crystalloids—A continuing controversy. Drug Intell Clin Pharm 18: 202–212, March 1984

Salter M: Towards a healthy body image. Nurs Mirror 157(11): ii–vi, September 14, 1983

Schneider J: The confused patient. Nurs Times 43–46, January 25, 1984

Schumann D: Preoperative measures to promote wound healing. Nurs Clin North Am 14(4): 683–699, December 1979

Schumann D: The nature of wound healing. AORN J 35(6): 1068–1077, May 1982

Schwartz RA, Cerra FB: Shock: A practical approach. Urol Clin North Am 10(1): 89–100, February 1983

Shapiro J, Hoffmann J, Jersky J: A comparison of suprapubic and transurethral drainage for postoperative urinary retention in general surgical patients. Acta Chir Scand 148(4): 323–327, 1982

Siskind J: Handling hemorrhage wisely. Nurs 84 14(1): 34–41, 1984

Smith CE: Detecting acute abdominal distension—What to look for, what to do. Nurs 85 15(9): 34–40, 1985

Smith DL: Septic shock. Top Emerg Med 5(2): 34–39, July 1983

Stock MC, Downs, JB, Gauer PK, Alster JM et al: Prevention of postoperative pulmonary complications with CPAP, incentive spirometry, and conservative therapy. Chest 87(2): 151–157, 1985

Stuhler–Schlag MK: Pre and postoperative fluids and electrolytes—Nursing assessment and intervention. Today's OR Nurse 4(7): 11–15, 66–67, September 1982

Sweeney SS: OR observations: Key to postop pain. AORN J 32(3): 391–400, September 1980

Taylor AG, West BA, Simon B, Skelton J et al: How effective is TENS for acute pain? Am J Nurs 83(8): 1171–1174, 1983

Taylor DL: Respiratory acidosis—Physiology, signs, and symptoms. Nurs 84 14(10): 44–45, 1984

Teasley KM, Lysne J, Nuwer N, Shronts EP et al: Nutrition and metabolic support of the surgical patient. Urol Clin North Am 10(1): 119–129, February 1983

Thomas MN: Acute pulmonary embolism. Focus Crit Care 10(4): 21–28, August 1983

Tulloch AGS: An algorithm for the management of postoperative urinary retention. Br J Surg 71(8): 638–639, 1984

Turpie AGG, Hirsch J: Venous thromboembolism: Current concepts—Part 1. Hosp Med 151–166, October 1984

Turpie AGG, Hirsh J: Venous thromboembolism: Current concepts—Part 2. Hosp Med 13–41, November 1984

Walts LF, Kaufman RD, Moreland JR, Weiskopf M: Total hip arthroplasty—An investigation of factors related to postoperative urinary retention. Clin Orthop (194): 280–282, April 1985

Wassner A: The impact of mutilating surgery or trauma on body-image. Int Nurs Rev 29(3): 86–90, May/June 1982

Warfield CA: Intraspinal narcotics. AORN J 41(5): 910–914, 1985

Wells N: The effect of relaxation on postoperative muscle tension and pain. Nurs Res 31(4): 236–238, July/August 1982

West BA: Understanding endorphins: Our natural pain relief system. Nurs 81 11(2): 50–53, 1981

Westaby S: Wound care No.1. Nurs Times: 77: September 23/29, 1981

Westaby S: Wound care No.3. Nurs Times 77: 9–12, November 18/24, 1981

Westaby S: Wound care No.4. Nurs Times 77: 13–16, December 16/22, 1981

Westaby S: Wound care No.6. Nurs Times 78: 21–24, February 17/23, 1982

Westaby S: Wound care No.7. Nurs Times 78: 25–28, March 17/23, 1982

Westaby S: Wound care No.8. Nurs Times 78: 29–32, April 21/27, 1982

Westaby S: Wound care No.9. Nurs Times 78: 33–36, May 19/25, 1982

Westra B: When your patient says "I can't breathe." Nurs 84 14(5): 34–39, 1984

Winters B: Promoting wound healing in the diabetic patient. AORN J 35(6): 1083–1088, May 1982

Wong ES: Guideline for Prevention of Catheter-Associated Urinary Tract Infections. Atlanta, U.S. Department of Health and Human Services Public Health Service Centers for Disease Control, 1981

Wright Z: From I.V. to P.O. Titrating your patient's pain medication. Nurs 81 7(11): 39–43, July 1981

Yasko JM: Holistic management of nausea and vomiting caused by chemotherapy. Top Clin Nurs 7(1): 26–38, April 1985

Yordan EL, Bernhard LA: The surgeon's role in wound healing. AORN J 35(6): 1078–1082, May 1982

9 | Discharge Planning

Discharge from the hospital or other health agency should never come unexpectedly to patients or to any of those attending them. The aim of the health team, patient, and the family, throughout the illness, is to make him or her independent. From the first, everyone should look forward to the day when the patient can leave the hospital.

—Virginia Henderson, Gladys Nite

The postoperative phase culminates in the patient's discharge from the hospital, either to home or to another health care facility. The nurse combines knowledge gleaned from the preoperative assessment with that relating to events of the intraoperative phase and plans for discharge with the patient and his family. Such discharge planning facilitates the smooth transition of care and ensures it continuity.

| The Goals of Discharge Planning

Discharge planning is a process by which the nurse identifies, with the patient and his family, those needs that must be met if the patient is to move smoothly from one level of care to another. By linking the patient and his family with resources that can meet identified needs, discharge planning ensures continuity of care, facilitates the progression of care from care by others to self-care, and promotes a patient's return to as normal and as productive a life as possible.

Discharge planning has always been a significant part of professional nursing practice. However, certain legislation has increased its importance and has necessitated changes in its structure. For example, Medicare has resulted not only in an increase in the number of hospitalizations for persons over age 65, but also in a decrease in the length of these hospitalizations. Diagnostic related groupings (DRGs) have contributed to shorter hospital stays. Postoperative patients are going home or to health care agencies with complex dressings and tubes to which they themselves, family members, or health care professionals must attend. In addition, many surgical procedures once requiring hospitalization for several days are now done in a one day surgery unit or on an outpatient basis.

The Discharge Planning Process

Assessment

The key to good discharge planning is early recognition of potential problems. Therefore, planning for a patient's discharge begins when he is admitted to the hospital. The nursing history, together with data provided by the physician on a Planning Assessment Guide (Figure 9-1), offers information about the total health care needs of the patient and his family. Additionally, the patient identifies with the nurse his strengths, limitations, problems, needs, and priorities. Together, they identify real or potential problems relating to his physical and emotional well-being, his learning needs, and the effects of hospitalization upon himself and his family.

Nursing Diagnosis

From the data collected, the nurse derives such nursing diagnoses as listed on page 266. The major diagnosis in this phase of the patient's perioperative experience relates to managing at home. However, other diagnoses, such as Self-care Deficit, are pertinent to discharge planning and were addressed earlier in the postoperative phase.

Once the diagnoses are derived, the nurse and patient together formulate corresponding goals. The nurse then devises a plan to meet these goals. Although the patient's discharge needs may change during hospitalization, information elicited upon admission enables the nurse to lay the groundwork for his discharge.

Planning

Just as the discharge planning process helps identify the patient's needs, so also it helps the nurse identify the health care professionals that need to be involved. Although the discharge planning process is a collaborative and multi-disciplinary effort, the nurse who works most closely with the patient and his family is the logical professional to coordinate the patient's care. The patient's needs determine whether the nurse and patient together can meet these needs or if other health care professionals need to be directly involved.

Patients with complex physical and social situations benefit from multi-

```
PLANNING ASSESSMENT GUIDE

Madison General Hospital
  202 South Park Street
  Madison, Wisconsin 53715
```

DATE	

(Complete upon admission. May update throughout hospital stay)

DIAGNOSIS:

ANTICIPATED LENGTH OF STAY: Days: ___1-3; ___4-6; ___7-10; ___more than 10

OBJECTIVE OF ADMISSION: (include major diagnostic studies, surgery, consults, etc.)

HEALTH TEACHING NEEDS: (___Teach Patient   ___Teach Family   ___Other)

   ___Medications   ___Wound Care   ___Equipment

   ___Nutrition/Diet   ___Disease Process   ___Resources

   ___Tests/Procedures ___None

   Comments:

POTENTIAL DISCHARGE PROBLEMS: ___None

   ___Multiple diagnoses   ___Alteration of body function

   ___Self-care deficits   ___Diet restriction

   ___Complicated Med/Rx regimen ___Chronic disease process

   ___Wound care   ___Inadequate support system (family/community)

   Comments: ___Psycho/Social Need

EXPECTED OUTCOME:

   ___No change of status   ___Surgery   ___Supportive care only

   ___Improved   ___Decreased function   (Indicate "No Code" order
                                                   on order sheet)

DESTINATION/REFERRALS: ___Alternative living arrangements

   ___Home, no assistance   ___Extended care facility

   ___Home, assistance needed   ___Visiting nurse   ___Other

PATIENT AND/OR FAMILY AWARE OF PLAN   ___Yes   ___No

Figure 9-1. Planning assessment guide. (Courtesy Madison General Hospital, Madison, WI)

disciplinary conferences. The patient's primary nurse attends these conferences, as do other health care professionals who have contributions to make to the patient's care plan.

The specific objectives to be met during such a conference are identified prior to it. Identification of the objectives facilitates their discussion at the conference. Objectives may relate to assessing a patient's personal needs, ensuring continuity of care by communicating with members of the health team, identifying specific needs of the patient and family, or devising a plan to meet the patient's special discharge needs. While neither feasible nor necessary

---

**Nursing Diagnosis Pertinent
to Discharge Planning**

Impaired home maintenance management related to lack of knowledge
about specifics of discharge plan

Self-care deficit related to appliances, prostheses, and assistive devices to
achieve self-care

From Kim MJ, McFarland GK, McLane AM (eds). Pocket Guide to Nursing Diagnoses. St. Louis, CV
Mosby, 1984

---

for all patients, multidisciplinary conferences can decrease the patient's anxiety about being discharged and facilitate a smooth transition, thus preventing problems and emergency admissions.

The Discharge Plan

All patients need a discharge plan. However, the specifics depend upon the patient's needs. Discharge plans run the gamut from providing information, to teaching the patient and his family to use equipment, to making a referral for home health care. Patient assessment factors considered in developing a discharge plan are outlined on page 267. These factors and others similar to them have been used to develop screening criteria that help identify patients needing specific discharge planning. The nursing history, initial preoperative patient assessment, and subsequent reassessments provide information about many of these factors.

Because the nurse orchestrates both the discharge planning process and the discharge plan, she develops a teaching-learning plan with the patient. (See the "Guidelines" on page 268.) When identifying his educational and learning needs, the nurse considers "generic" discharge planning items, that is, medications, diet, activity, treatments and procedures, signs and symptoms of potential complications, and return appointments. Depending upon the complexity of the patient's needs and her own knowledge, the nurse decides how best to meet the patient's discharge needs. She does some teaching herself and reinforces that done by other health care providers. Additionally, she may request referrals.

The nurse and other health care providers often use written materials as the basis for discharge planning. Written patient discharge instructions can pertain to specific aspects of the discharge plan such as medications (see the "Medication Guidelines" on page 270) or can include all aspects of the plan as illustrated in Figure 9-2. Written instructions provide the nurse with guidelines, and can be used to document teaching; the patient can also refer to them at home. However, written instructions do not eliminate the need for individual nurse-patient teaching.

Patient Assessment Factors To Be Considered in Developing a Discharge Plan

Physiologic Factors

General physical health and functional abilities

Disease processes

Surgical procedure performed

Patient's diagnosis

Current treatments and therapies

Current medications

General nutritional status

Diet, including food and fluids

Level of motor activity

Sensory awareness

Psychological Factors

Self-concept

Perceived level of well-being

Motivational strengths

Emotional functioning

Memory

Intelligence

Learning abilities

Social Factors

Internal social skills of the patient

Types of agency services required and available

Duration of care needed

Involvement of family in patient's care

Adapted from Shine, M.S.: **Discharge planning for elderly patient in the acute care setting.** Nurs Clin North Am 18(2): 403–410, June 1983

Documenting a patient's discharge plan facilitates its implementation and evaluation and therefore helps ensure continuity of care. Accurate and complete documentation is especially important when continuity among nursing staff is lacking.

Medication Instruction

Ideally, medication instruction is a cooperative effort among the patient, his family, the nurse, and the pharmacist. The purpose of the medication, proper

**Guidelines for Developing a
Teaching-Learning Plan**

Assess the patient's educational and learning needs. Keep in mind his cultural background and social class, which can affect his orientation to health.

Establish short- and long-term goals with the patient.

Develop instructional objectives and determine the patient's priorities in the learning process.

Ascertain the patient's current level of knowledge and his readiness to learn, including his motivation, attention span, stress level, developmental stage, and cognitive style.

Assess the patient's literacy level because this influences the type of instructional media used.

Select specific instructional strategies that facilitate attainment of the patient goals. These strategies should be varied and complement the patient's learning style.

Review educational media before using it. Consider the characteristics of the learner, the task, and the medium.

Select an environment conducive to learning, i.e., comfortable and free of distractions.

Keep teaching sessions short and periodically evaluate the teaching-learning process.

Begin each session with a brief review of the previous session.

When teaching a skill, ask the patient and, if appropriate, a family member or significant other, to return the demonstration.

Evaluate the overall effectiveness of patient teaching, including structure, process, and outcomes.

dosage and frequency, route, special instructions, potential side-effects, and occurrences that warrant notifying the physician are discussed.

Because the nurse spends the most time with the patient, she works with him and the pharmacist to establish a medication schedule that meshes with his life-style. Otherwise, the patient may leave the hospital thinking that he must take his medication according to the hospital schedule. If this schedule is unrealistic for him at home, he may stop taking the medication. Similarly, if the patient is to take a PRN medication, he must know and understand the criteria for self-medication.

In some hospitals the pharmacist does the initial teaching and the patient's nurse reinforces it. This approach means that the pharmacist and nurse must communicate. The nurse must know what the pharmacist told the patient. Otherwise, she may inadvertently give him conflicting information.

DISCHARGE INSTRUCTIONS

Madison General Hospital
Madison, Wisconsin

☐ No Diet Restrictions

DIET:

☐ No Medications

MEDICATIONS   DOSE   SCHEDULE   SPECIAL INSTRUCTIONS

☐ No Activity Restrictions

ACTIVITY:

☐ No Follow-up Appointments

FOLLOW-UP APPOINTMENT: DATE AND TIME   PHONE

PHYSICIAN'S SIGNATURE:

SPECIAL INSTRUCTIONS: DATE

COPY TO PATIENT: I HAVE READ AND UNDERSTAND THE ABOVE INSTUCTIONS
RN SIGNATURE: SIGNED:

711 - 63   814020   REV J 63

Figure 9-2. Discharge instructions. (Courtesy Madison General Hospital, Madison, WI)

And if confused, the patient may decide not to take his medication or to do so at his own discretion.

Frequently patients are given written medication instructions such as illustrated on page 270 for Digoxin. Several studies[1] indicate that written instructions when used *alone* do not improve a patient's compliance over a long period of time for taking medications prescribed. However, results indicate that written instructions frequently improve a patient's knowledge about precautions, side-effects, and special directions.

Medication Guidelines: Digoxin (Lanoxin)

What Digoxin Is Used for and How It Works

- Improves the ability of your heart to pump blood..
- Slows and regulates your heart rate.

How To Take Digoxin

- Take this medicine **exactly as directed** by your doctor even if you feel well.
- If you miss a dose of Digoxin, do not take the missed dose at all, and do NOT double the next one. Instead, go back to your regular schedule. If you have any questions, check with your doctor.
- Try to take this medicine at the same time every day to help you remember to take it.

Side-Effects of Digoxin

Along with its desirable effects, a medicine may cause some unwanted effects. Although not all of these effects appear very often, when they do occur, they may require medical attention. Check with your doctor if any of the following side effects occur:

Loss of appetite

Unusual tiredness or weakness

Lower stomach pain

Unusually slow or irregular pulse

Nausea or vomiting

Mental depression or confusion

Diarrhea

Special Instructions

- While you are taking Digoxin, check your pulse daily. If it is slower than _____ beats per minute, or if it changes in rhythm, check with your doctor.
- While you are on Digoxin, take only those medications, prescription and nonprescription, that have been okayed by your physician or pharmacist.
- This medicine may look like other tablets you take. **It is important that you do not get your medicines mixed up.**
- Although these symptoms may not be caused by Digoxin, notify your physician if you develop more shortness of breath, rapid weight gain, or increased swelling in your feet.

Additional Information

- Store Digoxin in a cool, dry place in the container you received from your pharmacy. The bathroom is not a good place because of dampness.
- Keep Digoxin out of the reach of children.
- Do not share your medicine with relatives or friends.

Numbers To Call If You Have Questions about or Problems with The Use of Digoxin

Dietary Instruction

If a specific diet has been prescribed for a patient, the nurse can request a dietary consult. By sharing the information that she gave the patient and his family, the dietitian enables the nurse to reinforce the teaching.

If a dietary consult is unavailable, the nurse herself teaches the patient about the diet. The nurse also includes in the teaching the person who will be doing the cooking. Together they can explore any implications that the diet may have for other family members and for the household budget. The patient and his family must understand not only the "what" of the diet, but also the "why" and "how."

Activity Instruction

Frequently the postoperative patient must limit physical activity for 4 to 6 weeks. The nurse explains the rationale for any restrictions and relates them specifically to the patient's life-style. For example, "no heavy lifting" may mean a laundry basket to one patient and 25 pounds of cement to another. Furthermore, the nurse explores the effect of these limitations upon the patient's life-style. Is it reasonable for the patient to comply with them? If not, what compromises can be made?

Treatments and Procedures

When teaching a patient to perform a treatment or procedure, the nurse uses clear, nontechnical language and includes a significant other in the teaching. Initially, they may only watch the nurse. But gradually, they become more involved, eventually doing the procedure several times before the patient's discharge.

Trying to anticipate problems that the patient may encounter at home, the nurse explains the importance of continuing the treatment and helps him modify it to fit his life-style. If a treatment requires certain equipment, a basin, for example, the nurse discusses with the patient equipment at home that he can use. Otherwise, the patient may think that he needs the exact same equipment and supplies as were used in the hospital.

Signs and Symptoms of Potential Complications

Length of hospital stay for surgical patients is decreasing, and many surgical procedures are performed in ambulatory care settings and one day surgery units. Therefore, patients need to know the signs and symptoms of potential postoperative complications that may develop at home. For example, since wound infections develop between the fifth and seventh postoperative day, the patient must know what to do if the incision becomes reddened, increasingly sore, or starts to drain, or if his temperature becomes elevated.

Other postoperative complications about which the patient needs information depend upon the procedure performed. For example, the patient who has a stoma needs to know that it should always be pink, moist, and visible. Similarly, if a patient were placed in the lithotomy position during surgery, he should be aware of the signs and symptoms of deep vein thrombosis. The nurse describes the signs and symptoms in a nonthreatening and nonalarming manner and instructs the patient to notify his physician immediately should they develop.

Return Appointments

A patient who is feeling well at home may decide not to keep his return appointment. Therefore, the nurse explains the importance of keeping such appointments and makes sure that the patient has the telephone number of the physician's office. The nurse also asks how the patient will get to the physician's office. She may need to explore community transportation resources such as bussing for the elderly and handicapped.

Referrals

The nurse begins thinking about the possible need for a referral when a patient is admitted. The nurse reassesses that possibility as she plans with the patient, his family, and physician for discharge. She defines the needs, based on the patient's physical, emotional, and psychosocial status. What are the specific needs of the patient and his family? How do they perceive the situation? What is being done about it now, and what will need to be done about it at home? Can what needs to be done, be done? For example, will the patient need Meals on Wheels? Does he need to go to an extended care facility or nursing home for 2 to 3 weeks before going home? Is the patient an alcoholic who wants to join Alcoholics Anonymous? If the nurse believes a referral would be helpful, she discusses her rationale with the patient and his family. The patient, however, ultimately makes the decision.

In most hospitals the patient's nurse initiates a referral. She contacts the home care coordinator or discharge planning nurse who is the liaison between the hospital and community agencies. Working together, the patient's nurse and the discharge planning nurse can ensure a smooth transition for the patient from hospital to home or other health care agency.

If the nurse herself *makes* the referral, she must be knowledgeable about community resources. Each agency has different goals and purposes, so when choosing an agency, the nurse considers the kind of services needed, the kind an agency provides, the agency's purpose, what can be expected of it, and its expectations of clients. If the agency requires a written referral, such as illustrated in Figure 9-3, the nurse and patient may be able to complete some sections together, that is, the patient care plan.

Some agencies have specific criteria regarding who can make the initial contact. For example, although a nurse can initiate a referral to Reach to Recovery, a physician's order is needed before the volunteer will visit a hospitalized patient.

Once the referral has been made, the nurse tells the patient what he can expect. For example, the visiting nurse will see him the first week at home on

Inter-Agency Nursing Referral Form

FORM PREPARED BY REPRESENTATIVES FROM HOSPITALS, NURSING HOMES & HEALTH AGENCIES
Courtesy of <u>DANE COUNTY PUBLIC HEALTH DEPARTMENT</u>   (241-4481)

Hospital Record No. _____   Date Called to Agency: _____

By: _____
(Name)   (Unit)

TO: _____ FROM: _____
(Name of Hospital or Nursing Home)

PATIENT NAME _____ Telephone No. _____
(First)   (M.I.)   (Last)

Address: _____

Directions: _____

Birthdate: ____/____/____ Date Admitted: _____ Date Discharged: _____

Significant Other: _____ Relationship: _____

REPORT FROM ATTENDING PHYSICIAN

Diagnosis: _____ Prognosis: _____

Additional Diagnoses: _____

PHYSICIAN'S ORDERS:
   Medications: _____   _____

   _____   _____

   _____   _____

   _____   _____

   _____   _____

   _____   _____

   Treatments: _____

   _____

Level of Activity: _____ Mental Status: _____

Diet: _____ Safety Concerns: _____

Rehabilitation Potential: _____ Supplies or Appliances Needed: _____

Functional Limitations: _____

Type of Services Ordered: (Please Check)
☐ Nursing/Health Aide   ☐ Physical Therapy Evaluation & Service   ☐ Occupational Therapy Evaluation & Service
☐ Social Service Counseling   ☐ Speech Therapy

I CERTIFY THIS PATIENT IS ESSENTIALLY HOMEBOUND AND REQUIRES SKILLED NURSING CARE: ☐ Yes   ☐ No

Estimated Length of Time Services Needed: _____

PHYSICIAN'S SIGNATURE _____ **DATE:** _____

Attach Reports from Dietician, Medical Social Worker, Physical Therapist, Occupational Therapist, Speech Therapist.
231-61-10 (4/83)   (continued)

Figure 9-3. Interagency nursing referral form (A and B). Prepared by representatives from hospitals, nursing homes, and health agencies. (Courtesy Dane County WI, Public Health Department)

Monday, Wednesday, and Friday to help him manage his colostomy appliance.

Sometimes referrals are made to an agency that the patient must visit, for example, social welfare or vocational rehabilitation agencies. In such situations, the nurse makes sure the patient knows the location of the agency and if

NURSING CARE PLAN

PAST HISTORY (medical/surgical, sight, hearing, etc.)	HISTORY OF PRESENT ILLNESS (interventions)	

TREATMENT (patient/family teaching, proficiency; supplies-given/needed; etc.)	PSYCHOSOCIAL (patient/family responses)	MEDICATIONS (Patient understanding, patient/family teaching)	
		DATE OF SURGERY:	
		VS:	ALLERGIES:
		DIET:	WEIGHT:
	SPECIFIC PROBLEMS (suggested approach, referrals, etc.)	ACTIVITY LEVEL:	
		SAFETY CONCERNS:	
		ADL'S:	
		ELIMINATION:	
		EQUIPMENT:	
		OTHER AGENCIES INVOLVED:	

Nurse's Signature _____ Title _____ Date _____

PUBLIC HEALTH AGENCY REPORT (Home situation, special problems, evidence of progress, how is patient progressing, and result of public health intervention). Date of first home visit following referral _____ .

I plan to continue to visit: ☐ Yes ☐ No

Signature _____ Title _____ Date _____

Form prepared by representatives from hospitals, nursing homes and health agencies (Dane County)
Printing — Courtesy of **DANE COUNTY PUBLIC HEALTH DEPARTMENT**

possible, gives him the name of a contact person. The nurse also tells him what to expect during the first visit, how long he may have to wait, and what documents he will need to present. She anticipates as many of the potential barriers as possible, but the patient makes the final decision whether or not to keep the appointment.

The Discharge Summary

A discharge summary is much more than a sentence stating, "Patient discharged to home with family." It is a concise synopsis that highlights the events of a patient's hospitalization and is completed when the patient is discharged. Outlining the patient's hospitalization, his condition, and treatment, the summary can be used when making a referral and may take one of four forms: source-oriented, problem-oriented, checklist, or a combination of these.

The source-oriented system and the problem-oriented patient record present the same information but in different formats. The source-oriented system uses a narrative style, while the problem-oriented record highlights certain aspects of information. Either the acronym SOAP or SOAPIER is used. "S" refers to subjective data, including the patient's description of his symptoms. "O" includes objective data such as the patient's vital signs and other information obtained via observation and examination. The letter "A" notes the assessment or conclusion of the patient's problem and "P" identifies the plan for the patient. Intervention, noted with an "I", describes therapies already initiated, while evaluation, "E", delineates the outcome of the interventions. The letter "R" indicates revisions or alterations made in the plan.

Checklists or printed discharge slips may be adequate for recording discharge summaries. If space on the checklist is inadequate, other sheets of paper can be added. Each page is numbered sequentially and the patient's name, hospital number, and the date and time are written at the top of each successive page.

Evaluation

The patient and his family are prepared for discharge and the continuity of the patient's care is ensured.

Summary

Working with a patient and his family from admission to discharge, the professional nurse establishes a therapeutic relationship with them. She sees the patient as the unique individual he is, with specific needs, problems, and goals. Because she knows both the patient's needs and community resources, the nurse is able to help the patient make a smooth transition from one level of care to another. Outcome criteria relevant to discharge planning are listed on page 276.

**Outcome Criteria for a
Patient Being Discharged**

1. The patient correctly describes the specifics of his discharge plan,
   including medication, dietary and activity instruction, signs and
   symptoms of potential complications, and return appointments, and
   correctly demonstrates treatments and procedures.
2. The patient correctly demonstrates the use of assistive devices needed
   for self-care.

References

1. Morris LA, Halperin JA: Effects of written drug information on patient knowl-
    edge and compliance: A literature review. Am J Public Health 69(1): 47–52,
    1979

Bibliography

Baumgartner RG: Patient care conferencing. Crit Care Nurse 5(3): 59–65, May/June
    1985
Bayer M: Saying goodbye through graffitti. Am J Nurs 80(2): 271, 1980
Beale PP, Gulley MI: Discharge planning process: An interdisciplinary approach. Milit
    Med 146(1): 713–716, October 1981
Broomfield S: Involving staff in discharge planning. Supervisor Nurse 10(7): 35–38,
    1979
Chisholm MM: Promises and pitfalls of discharge planning. Nurs Mgmt 14(11):
    26–29, 1983
Clausen C: Staff RN: A discharge planner for every patient. Nurs Mgmt 15(11):
    58–61, 1984
Connolly ML: Organize your workday for more effective discharge planning. Nurs 81
    11(7): 44–47, 1981
Cunningham LS: Early assessment for discharge planning. Qual Rev Bull October:
    11–16, 1981
Filandro DV: Discharge planning: Presenting the case. Nurs Mgmt 14(11): 17–18,
    1983
Gikow F, Anderson E, Bigelow L, Bossi L, et al: The continuing care nurse. Nurs
    Outlook 33(4): 195–197, July/August 1985
Glover JC: Reducing discharge planning paperwork with a pocket-size discharge plan-
    ning record. Nurs 81 11(12): 50–51, 1981
Habeeb MC, McClaughlin FE: Including the hospital staff nurse. Am J Nurs 79(8):
    1443–1445, 1979
Kim MJ, McFarland GK, McLane AM (eds): Pocket Guide to Nursing Diagnoses. St.
    Louis, CV Mosby, 1984
Morris LA, Halperin JA: Effects of written drug information on patient knowledge
    and compliance: A literature review. Am J Public Health 69(1): 47–52, 1979
Rasmussen LA: A screening tool promotes early discharge planning. Nurs Mgmt
    15(5): 39–43, 1984

Redman BK: The Process of Patient Education, 5th ed. St. Louis, CV Mosby, 1984

Reichelt PA, Newcomb J: Organizational factors in discharge planning. J Nurs Adm 10(12): 36–42, 1980

Reilly MA: Let's set the record straight. Nurs 79 9(1): 56–61, 1979

Romano CA: A computerized approach to discharge care planning. Nurs Outlook 32(1): 23–25, January/February 1984

Shine MS: Discharge planning for the elderly patient in the acute care setting. Nurs Clin North Am 18(2): 403–410, June 1983

Stone M: Discharge planning guide. Am J Nurs 79(8): 1446–1447, 1979

Wells MI: Discharge planning: Closing the gaps in continuity of care. Nurs 83 13(11): 45, 1983

Wheeler-Lachowycz J: How to use your VNA. Am J Nurs 83(8): 1164–1167, 1983

Index

Numbers followed by an *f* indicate a figure; *t* following a page number indicates tabular material.